Extraordinary Healing

How the discoveries of
Mirko Beljanski, the world's
first green molecular biologist,
can protect and restore
your health

by
L. Stephen Coles, M.D., Ph.D.

D1566284

Disclaimer: This information is presented by an
independent medical expert whose sources of information
include studies from the world's medical and scientific
literature, patient records, and other clinical and case
reports. The material in this book is for informational
purposes only and is not intended for the diagnosis,
treatment, cure or prevention of disease. Please visit a
health professional for medical advice or to discuss
information contained in this book.

Book design by Bonnie Lambert

ISBN 978-1-893910-89-8
Printed in the United States
Published by Freedom Press
120 North Topanga Canyon Boulevard
Topanga, CA 90290
Bulk Orders Available: (800) 959-9797
E-mail: info@freedompressonline.com

"Man in all its humanity has the duty not to conform but to fight the enemy of free thinking and to remain truthful to his own ideal as opposed to his clan."
—Erasmus, *The Praise of Folly*

"Industry is the livelihood of a civilized nation…but this industry that puts everything in motion, that enlivens society, borrows its strength from a primal source culled from sciences."
—Antoine Lavoisier, *Oeuvres*, T. IV p. 616

"Men who dedicate their life to the supreme art of making discoveries must be independent and free, their support must be warranted by the whole society. Do not demand of them that they teach, but let them create and publish because true discoveries are rare."
—Antoine Lavoisier, Rapport sur l'instruction publique présenté à la tribune de la Convention, circa 1793
(Lavoisier was guillotined on May 8, 1794)

Contents

Foreword

This book is foremost a story of hope and extraordinary perseverance. A founder of modern environmental medicine, Mirko Beljanski devised a revolutionary way of identifying early biomarkers or indicators of carcinogenic risk and became one of the world's first green molecular microbiologists. Fortunately, today, the practical applications of his findings are being studied and confirmed and made available to consumers around the world, providing prevention and support to patients affected with a number of serious illnesses.

Mirko Beljanski was both a hero of modern liberal society and a leader in the fields of medicine and biology. By saving the French president's life in 1995, he also influenced history at a time when the country was debating joining the European Union. In his adopted homeland of France, Mirko faced terrible oppression as conventional scientists rejected his revolutionary ideas about nutrition and the immune system. After a quarter of a century, he produced well over a hundred major peer-reviewed papers working with Nobel Laureates and other prize-winning scientists at the Pasteur Institute in Paris. What did Dr. Beljanski discover? He was perhaps the first to show how the environment speaks to our cells via a type of ribonucleic acid called reverse transcriptase (he was also first to discover this in bacteria and higher life forms). Basically, reverse transcriptase provides the capacity of RNA to communicate with the outside world, the environment, and that brings back messages to the cell that are taken up and transformed into our basic genetic material—our DNA. Mirko discovered that certain RNA fragments can actually induce the body to maintain healthy levels of platelets during even the most stressful times, and figured out how to apply this to clinical treatments.

Starting in 1972, by examining the physical structure of DNA, he also showed us that mutations are not one of the first, but one of the later, stages of cancer. He was able to show us pictures of the exquisite double helix as it is damaged and destabilized earlier.

Because his work challenged traditional approaches to oncology and medicine, Mirko was rejected and attacked by those working for the French pharmaceutical industry. Mirko recognized the importance of nutrition and infection for some forms of cancer and rejected the prevailing approach that relied on highly toxic drugs to kill cancer cells. The idea of boosting the immune system as a way to enhance the body's capacity to overcome cancer and other chronic diseases, as Mirko suggested, was dismissed by most commercial interests at the time.

A number of his concepts and ideas in the area of cancer treatment and prevention have found new support in contemporary research in immunology, bacteriology and oncology, and are now part of the vanguard of the greening of modern environmental medicine

Fortunately, the work of Dr. Beljanski has found a home in America where it is being actively investigated at the Columbia University Center for Holistic Urology. Some of the specific plant fragments he discovered have been shown to strongly inhibit errant cell growth and help the body to maintain a normal inflammation response. In addition, researchers such as Dr. Donald Malins, writing in the June 2006 *Environmental Health Perspectives* and other journals, have found subtle biochemical markers of damage and alterations that occur long before direct mutations are evident.

All of this adds up to an exciting and life-changing line of research by giving us new molecular tools with which to combat cancer, boost the immune system and reverse signs of disease before they advance to less treatable stages.

In the end, the insights of Dr. Mirko Beljanski have laid the foundation for a fundamental shift in how we approach diseases and wellness consistent with a number of cutting-edge researchers today. Mirko established an important, innovative approach to disease prevention and health promotion.

In this book, Dr. L. Stephen Coles has used his considerable experience in the fields of longevity medicine and natural health to bring us the incredible story of these important findings. Tens of thousands of people exposed to toxic chemicals from the workplace, the environment or from undergoing stressful periods of their lives due to these chemicals (including chemotherapy and radiation treatment) will benefit from his discoveries.

— Devra Lee Davis, Ph.D., Author, *Disconnect—The Truth About Cell Phone Radiation*; and *The Secret History of the War on Cancer*, and Visiting Professor, Georgetown University

The Father of Modern Environmental Medicine

The history of science is filled with stories of men and women who, with the truths that they have discovered, have challenged powerful interests. These heroes of science, politics and other realms of society often demonstrate great courage to face off against extremely well-funded, established and profitable cartels like the intertwined interests of the chemical and food industries and the cancer and medical establishment. These mavericks frequently suffer greatly for their courage to advocate truth, however unpopular and unwanted it may be—at least by the most powerful monied interests.

Galileo Galilei, the Tuscan physicist, mathematician, astronomer and philosopher who was born in 1564 and died in 1642, played a major role in the scientific revolution. Galileo's astronomical observation that the Earth, in fact, was not the center of the universe was so controversial during his life that the Catholic Church prohibited the advocacy of his heliocentrist theory. He was forced to recant heliocentrism and spent the last years of his life under house arrest on orders of the Catholic Inquisition.

Ignaz Philipp Semmelweis, born in 1818, was an Austrian-Hungarian physician known as the "savior of mothers." He discovered, by 1847, that the incidence of puerperal fever could be drastically cut by implementing hand-washing standards in obstetrical clinics. Puerperal fever (or childbed fever) was common in mid-19th century hospitals and often fatal, with mortality as high as 35 percent.

Semmelweis postulated the theory of washing with chlorinated lime solution in 1847 as head of Vienna General Hospital's First Obstetrical Clinic, where doctor wards had three times the mortality of midwife wards. By 1861, despite his published findings of statistically significant clinical trials showing hand washing reduced mortality below 1 percent, Semmelweis' practice only earned widespread acceptance years after his death, when Louis Pasteur confirmed the germ theory.

In *The Secret History of the War on Cancer*, Devra Lee Davis, Ph.D., former director of the University of Pittsburgh Environmental Oncology Center and one of the world's leading cancer epidemiologists, tells how following World War II, the great industrial doctor and scientist Wilhelm Hueper, while working for DuPont, discovered that the benzidine dyes the company produced were causing occupational cancers. The company suppressed his work and prohibited him from ever visiting its industrial plants again. Hueper then went to work for the recently formed National Cancer Institute but instead of being allowed to pursue his work, he was persecuted and branded as a communist, again because of the inordinate industry pressure from without and within the NCI.

It's the way of doing people in. It's a blood sport. Like Hueper, many people— particularly crusaders—hold the truth in high regard. But when it is inconvenient, the truth is often the last thing powerful petrochemical, medical, pharmaceutical and agricultural interests want to hear.

Dr. Davis could not have written her momentous work had she remained at the National Academy of Sciences. Her decision to leave the NAS afforded her the freedom to write one of the most important contemporary historic works on cancer today.

Contemporaneously, Chris Delarosa endured persecution by the Agency of Toxic Substances Disease Registry (ATSDR) for advising Hurricane Katrina survivors to leave their formaldehyde-contaminated trailers provided by the Federal Emergency Management Agency. He lost his position at the ATSDR because he advocated prudence. Despite being punished for telling the truth about the unhealthy government-issued trailers, Delarosa's actions helped make millions of consumers aware of the formaldehyde-tainted trailers.

The truth does come to light eventually; often due to the selfless efforts of a courageous few who pursue truth for the good of the many.

Mirko Beljanski, Ph.D., was one such scientist. He spent a quarter century conducting controversial research at the Pasteur Institute where the Institute's director, Jacques Monod, suppressed his work in an epic battle to defend the primacy of cellular DNA over RNA. This is, in a sense, a "war story" worth telling.

Today, Beljanski's discovery showing that destabilized deoxyribonucleic acid (DNA) is at the heart of cancer causation is critical to the development of selective nontoxic treatments for cancer and new and important methods of chemical toxicity screening. And so too are his findings that RNA remakes DNA.

Medical doctors throughout Europe and North America are now using these treatments based on Beljanski's molecules to help millions of people stay healthy. It's time for the public to know about Beljanski's approach to complementary medicine.

Beljanski's work is currently enjoying a renaissance because major institutions have taken it up and are studying its efficacy. The growing acceptance of his theories by researchers at powerful institutions like Columbia University and the Cancer Treatment Centers of America could help Beljanski's methods become the backbone of complementary medicine and an accepted way of viewing cellular damage for screening purposes.

Indeed, his findings are rapidly infiltrating the mainstream. It is as if he is more alive now than ever. Beljanski's fundamental research and its scientific dissemination may finally help the global health community in its fight to win the war on cancer.

As Beljanski's findings are detailed and explored, these fundamental ideas are sure to influence the scientific views of experts and lead to a whole new class of chemicals being identified as early carcinogens or what some experts think of as pro-carcinogens or cancer promoters—chemicals that cause cumulative damage to the cellular structure, independently of genetic mutations. Mutations tell only a small part of the story and may well be a consequence of DNA destabilization, which is what makes cells susceptible to reproducing too much of what we call cancer.

Beljanski's contributions in the field of molecular biology, while known in his own time and appreciated by European doctors, immunology experts, and other clinicians, were particularly controversial in his beloved France, where its leading scientists were focused entirely on the mutational theory of cancer—and winning the Nobel Prize! The story of Nobel Prize winner Jacques Monod and Beljanski, both of whom were scientific foes at the Pasteur Institute, is a classic one.

Monod, native to France, was the director of the department where Beljanski was working, and later, of the entire Pasteur Institute and his chief nemesis—in what truly was a battle of epic scientists who both believed they had discovered an important secret of nature.

Mirko's findings challenged the basic orthodoxy of genetic research that was centered on the primacy of cellular DNA as the ultimate director of humankind's biological and genetic fate.

From Monod, a Huguenot, Beljanski faced enormous opposition. Monod was hardheaded and unyielding with his belief in the omnipotence of DNA. Indeed, it was Monod who engineered Beljanski's demise within the highly competitive world of the Pasteur Institute, though Monod steadfastly denied wrongdoing to the end.

But it wasn't just Monod. That was only one level of persecution, and frankly, if Beljanski had faced Monod alone, he would have thrived nonetheless, perhaps in another lab funded by more independent thinkers who saw the potential in his work. The most dangerous attacks, however, came from the medical establishment, even after he treated the French President and prolonged his life, despite the nature of his cancer. But, again, these attacks emanated from his foes at the Pasteur Institute. Together, they savagely dogged Beljanski. Sadly, for the rest of the world, the medical bureaucracy, Monod and his allies in France successfully suppressed Beljanski's work for decades even though it offered potentially life-saving help. Most tragically, Beljanski was indicted, subjected to illicit search and seizure, and set to be put on trial without a date in violation of his basic human rights.

Despite this shameful chapter in French history, one can only hope for the sake of the French people that the Beljanski molecules receive their just due throughout France and Europe, thanks to the work of American scientists who've championed his work.

Beljanski was a man who saw what others abstracted. He saw the three-dimensional change of the DNA structure. By his way of seeing things with the use of melting point and spectrophotometry, he highlighted the damaging effects of chemicals on the conformational structure of DNA before or without mutations in the genes. *Mutations in the DNA might appear, only later, since they are facilitated by DNA destabilization and by then, it is often too late to reverse the damage.*

In fact, with more than 130 peer-reviewed scientific publications, Beljanski's contributions are being belatedly recognized as major contributions to the field of environmental medicine.

With the help of the Beljanski plant molecules and RNA fragments, people throughout Europe and increasingly also in the United States who are following his scientific findings are enjoying long lives of good quality. To seize a brighter future, it is imperative that we learn about healing the double helix and the very secrets of life that Beljanski discovered.

Part I
Mirko's
Discovery

———— ～～～～ ————

October 9, 1996

In the heart of France in the Rhone Valley, there are small, peaceful villages sleeping in the sun. On the eastern bank of the river, the heavy grape bunches ripen in the vineyards, which will soon give generous wines with prestigious names: Côte Rôtie, Crozes-Hermitage, St. Joseph, Chateau-Grillet.... They are divine with duck or the like.

On the western bank, nestled in a small valley, there are other quiet villages. One of them is called St. Prim. In the olden days, the manor of St. Prim, a beautiful property dating back to the beginning of the 19th century, belonged to the Pomerol family who, in addition to their vineyards in the Bordeaux region, also owned numerous nearby vineyards. In the 1960s, the family abandoned the residence, which was put on the market. In the ensuing years, weather and lack of upkeep had damaged it and depreciated its value. This is how CIRIS (the Centre d'Innovations, de Recherches et d'Informations Scientifiques), a not-for-profit organization dedicated to the advancement of medical and scientific research with no political agenda, was able to acquire it for a relatively modest price. Thanks to the work of local AIDS patients who were hoping that the work of CIRIS might offer them hope, the property was renovated and made beautiful.

The former horse stable was transformed into a modern scientific laboratory where a team of five to seven scientists and technicians worked. This serene environment was perfect to reflect and think. Mirko Beljanski, an aging man and the head of this small team, was putting the finishing touches on his novel experiments that were leading to breakthroughs in cancer research. He loved the rou-

20   •   Extraordinary Healing

tine of working in his lab and going for walks in the park. It was perfect for Mirko's scientifically creative mindset. After a quarter century at the prestigious Pasteur Institute, Mirko was a free man—or so he believed.

Then, on October 9, 1996, early in the morning, a column of seven or eight police cars filled with security agents carrying weapons zeroed in on St. Prim. It was the Groupe d'Intervention de la Gendarmerie Nationale (GIG), an elite French police detachment used in high-risk operations. They blocked all roads to regular traffic. Villagers observed with great surprise this strange scene that clashed with the normally peaceful environment.

The armed forces crawled toward the building, cut the fences surrounding the park, and finally entered the premises. The plan was to surprise the residents who were still asleep at that early hour. At 7 a.m., all hell broke loose: Doors were forced open, the dogs barked vociferously and ferociously, and police, security agents and canines invaded the building. The police ordered everyone outside. They had come to arrest Mirko Beljanski. They confiscated his lab equipment, removed his notebooks, and took away his team. They handcuffed the scientist and loaded three trucks with his equipment before driving him to the train station and putting him under high surveillance on a train to Paris. Employees were stunned.

Nobody understood. Why ransack his lab? Who was this scientist named Mirko Beljanski?

CHAPTER ONE

Paris

Mirko Beljanski was born on March 27, 1923, to a family of farm workers in the poor Serbian village of Turija in the north of Serbia in the Vojvodina province. The region was, and still is, devoted to corn, farm animals, and sunflowers.

Despite Turija's 6,000 residents, the village did not have a store. Its large unpaved roads were muddy when it rained and dusty as soon as it dried. Houses made of mud or bricks with colored wash gave a lively and joyful look to those long roads, all perpendicular and identical. The community well was 200 meters from the house—and it was the only source of water around. Turija had no electricity, cars or paved roads until the 1980s. The village has long had a Serb ethnic majority. It is most famous, of course, for its annual sausage festival known as *Kobasicijada*.

The mud floor of Mirko's childhood home was covered with coarsely multicolored, handloom-woven cloth. Despite the difficulties of life, everything was perfectly clean. Like so many other children in Turija, Mirko played European football with a frenzy. Before long, however, his carefree demeanor gave way to the realities of his family's persistent and oppressive financial problems. Mirko's father was a smalltime iron worker who repaired wheeled carriages, wells, and harvesting machines.

While most of his peers planned to follow in their father's footsteps, Mirko had other plans. He wanted to create—though he did not know what yet. He was driven to accomplish. Since infancy, Mirko had longed to go to primary school with his two older sisters. As a teenager, he made it clear that he wanted to study at a lyceum (secondary school) and escape the surrounding fatalism of this village deep in the heart of the former Yugoslavia.

Study was the only way. But at that time, it was very unusual for children to go to high school: There were only two children in this village of 6,000 who could pursue higher education. His father also did not want him to leave Turija for the lyceum, as he wanted his son to learn his trade and help him. They argued. In the end, his father lost, as fathers often do when they argue with their children.

The lyceum was 30 to 40 miles away in a town called Novi Sad. Despite the cost and his father's resistance, his mother and two older sisters (who were seamstresses) managed to enroll him in the lyceum. Kissing his mother's cheek and hugging his father and sisters, 12-year-old Mirko said goodbye to his family and village forever.

EARLY EDUCATION

Novi Sad is Serbia's second-largest city, after Belgrade. In its most recent official census from 2002, the city had an urban population of 216,583, while its municipal population was 299,294. The city is located on the border of the Bačka and Syrmia regions, on the banks of the Danube river and Danube-Tisa-Danube Canal, facing the northern slopes of Fruška Gora mountain.

In Novi Sad, Mirko spent four years with an uncle without children, and thereafter four years with an aunt. The first year seemed very difficult for the young rough peasant. Although he missed his family, he persevered and the following years were easier.

Throughout these years, Mirko did not exhibit a marked taste for science. He worked hard to fill the gaps that his humble origins brought to his education. He was an extremely good observer, very self-educated and disciplined.

When he received his general certificate (baccalaureate), his school also presented him with a special gift (a gold coin) to reward his efforts. Unfortunately, war broke out the very same year he finished school, dividing his country faced with both a civil war and the German invasion. Some fought against the Germans, while others, fueled by the fear of communism, made an alliance with Germany to fight the partisans of the resistance. Mirko felt an urgency to fight the German invasion, and joined the partisans until the end of the war.

When the war ended, he received two educational offers from the Yugoslavian government that had been arranged for him. He could go either to Moscow or Paris. It wasn't a tough choice.

He was sent to Paris with a two-year fellowship from the French Foreign Office. He arrived in Paris during a rainy day in autumn 1945. He still knew very little French and immediately, with untamed determination that would never fail him, he enrolled at La Sorbonne (Faculté of Sciences) where he discovered what would be his passion for life—biology, biochemistry, and the wonderful complexity and sophistication of the biological world.

With no family support and just a small grant, life was difficult. He had very little money to pay for his narrow, inexpensive room under the roof in a small hotel located in the 14th arrondissement (a Paris district), near the Cité Universitaire where he had dinner, while courses were given in the Latin Quarter at the Sorbonne. Mirko did what he was used to: doing as much as he could in the minimum amount of time. He had a single objective and focused on it. He was not interested in politics, because when he was in Yugoslavia during the civil war, he became aware that war and politics bring only destruction and hatred. "Because of Mirko's sensitivity and his taste," said his wife Monique Beljanski, "he focused on the beauty of the biological world which, contrary to human passion, was more predictable and logical."

Mirko concluded his studies just as his grant ran out. He was obliged to return to Yugoslavia where he worked for five months in a lab in Belgrade. Then he was lucky enough to receive another grant from the World Health Organization, and he returned to Paris. In 1949, he joined the prestigious Pasteur Institute in the Department of Chemical Biology, headed by Michel Macheboeuf, to prepare his doctorate.

It was a wonderful yet dark time in the field of genetic science. Molecular biology had not yet been born and neither DNA nor its structure envisioned.

As recently as 1930, DNA was considered to be a cellular buffer, because of its high content in phosphate. Few scientists were focused on DNA or RNA in relation to protein synthesis.

Nobody conceived then of the tiny back and forth messaging from within the complex structure inside each cell. In Brussels (Belgium), the embryologist Jean Brachet (1909-1988) was one of the first scientists to be interested in DNA and RNA. Through cytochemical methods, he demonstrated the presence of both nucleic acids in all mammalian cells, and in particular, those that have a high level of protein synthesis. In his own words memorialized in a 1987 symposium proceeding, Brachet recalled, "I had of course read and reread the few pages that books on biochemistry dedicated to nucleic acids. They all stated that there exist two types (true): thymus nucleic acid in animals and zymonucleic acid in plants. The first one (DNA) has a mysterious sugar, deoxyribose, and the second one (RNA) a classical pentose, ribose…. A rash and false generalization had led to the conclusion that DNA was an 'animal' nucleic acid and RNA was a 'vegetal' nucleic acid."[1]

Early observations had led him to a quite different view and finally he found that sea urchin eggs did contain large amounts of pentoses, mostly in the form of RNA. Thus, Brachet had exposed as a myth that RNA was only of vegetal origin.

"After several not very encouraging attempts, I found in 1939 a simple cytochemical technique for detecting RNA in cells," continued Brachet. "To my great joy, I found RNA, like DNA, to be a universal constituent of cells—bacterial, vegetal, and animal. The intracellular localization of these two types of nucleic acid is, however, quite different: whereas DNA is found in chromatin and chromosomes, RNA accumulates in cytoplasm and nucleoli." Then he added something spectacularly important that would also compel Mirko's own future direction in research. "In addition, whereas the amount of DNA per nucleus remains constant in a particular species (allowing for its doubling when cells prepare for division), the amount of RNA varies considerably from one tissue to another; I saw a completely unexpected correlation between the quantity of RNA in a cell and its capacity to synthesize proteins. This led me to another iconoclastic proposition: Proteins are not synthesized by proteolytic enzymes operating backwards, as was generally thought, but by an unknown mechanism implicating RNA. The same conclusion was arrived at simultaneously (1941) by T. Caspersson in Stockholm, who was using a completely different technique for the cytochemical detection of nucleic acids."

During the late 19th and early 20th centuries, organic chemistry was the focus of research in Germany. German science was highly regarded in France. However, that all ended with World War II and the German occupation; at that time there was a break in the relationships with the Anglo-Saxon world. During the German occupation, England and the United States were developing a new approach to science with all of the latest scientific equipment, including gas chromatography and mass spectrometry, while France could not afford to modernize its scientific equipment and had very little contact with the outside world. (Most French scientists did not even speak English!)

But much of the problem was simply one of resources. France was lagging behind because of the war and the German occupation. Laboratories were old and poorly equipped. The central government had too much to rebuild and could not dedicate much financial support to the modernization of lab equipment.

"After four years of German occupation, laboratories were very poor," Monique recalled. "As a result, scientific research was behind. Young researchers had to spend a lot of their precious time to wash their tools, prepare reagents, and isolate enzymes, in addition to building their own equipment in many instances. (For example, Mirko learned how to blow glass.) There was no spectrophotometer, so much of the dosages were done by colorimetric reactions. On the other hand, these difficulties forced the scientists to learn new techniques, learn more about chemicals and their interactions, and how to control each reagent, which, in the end, turned out to be very useful training."

Naturally there was a tremendous interest at Pasteur in germ theory. Pasteur himself had demonstrated the power of microscopic organisms to cause illness, which led to the development of tiny poisons that could kill or subdue them, usually made from the metabolic byproducts of other bacteria or fungal organisms, now known as antibiotics, such as penicillin. But these same bacteria that antibiotics once killed were already beginning to show signs of outwitting the doctors' tools, and scientists wanted to know why.

Only a few years had elapsed since the first antibiotics appeared, yet there was already an acute awareness of bacterial antibiotic resistance. Why and how were certain germs or certain mutants coming from more sensitive strains able to resist the action of an antibiotic and become resistant? How did this evolution occur?

As a subject for his thesis, Macheboeuf, the head of the Department of Chemical Biology at Pasteur, suggested that Mirko study the origin of bacterial resistance to streptomycin. The young researcher had an idea he wished to prove: that several antibiotics were capable of inducing modifications in bacterial nucleic acids. In fact, he demonstrated that during the acquisition of resistance to antibiotics (streptomycin, penicillin and others...), the surviving bacteria kept accumulating RNA as opposed to wild bacteria that never met up with the antibiotics. Again we come back to what would be a central theme in Mirko's work: rather than DNA playing an exclusive role, RNA also seems to be a factor especially in antibiotic resistance, as RNA accumulates and "talks" to the environment, assesses it and makes genetic changes it will later take to the DNA, as indicated by its increased accumulation during the most excitable, adaptive, and changeable periods of life. Although Beljanski was among the first to become aware of the interaction between RNA and DNA, this phenomenon would later be confirmed by chemists completely unrelated and unaware of Beljanski's research.[2] Furthermore, these scientists determined that RNAs accumulated by the resistant bacteria are much richer in puric acid bases guananine and adenine (G and A).

From this discovery, Mirko developed the subject of his doctoral thesis, "Study of bacterial strains resistant to antibiotics: Compared to susceptible strains of the same species." Of course, there was much more he would learn that he would not understand until a decade later. Mirko carried out his research on bacterial antibiotic resistance for another three years until he completed his doctoral degree. This research allowed him to select the analytic methods that were to become essential in his subsequent DNA and RNA work and to begin new investigations of bacteria, which was his first step on the road to his later discoveries.

When his grant ended, Mirko would have to leave France and his work. Macheboeuf wrote a letter to the Minister of Public Health of the Yugoslavian Government asking to keep Mirko in France.

On June 25, 1951, Macheboeuf wrote, "In order to carry out his research, some special and complicated equipment is needed, which we have in my laboratory. If Mr. Beljanski leaves immediately for Yugoslavia, he will need to abandon his research (for which he is acclaimed), which would be a shame.

"Consequently, I am taking it upon myself, Mr. Minister, to ask you if you can consider an extension of Mr. Beljanski's stay in France. I was very happy to welcome into my laboratory this young Yugoslav of great worth, and I offer him my hospitality and servicing as long as he wants to pursue the magnificent research that he is undertaking."

Thanks to the letter that his superior wrote, Mirko was allowed to stay in France and complete his thesis. He published several articles whose conclusions showed that during the acquisition of resistance to different antibiotics, bacteria accumulated RNAs.

From then on, his interest in the different roles that RNAs play in the cells would never cease. Later, he would return to these topics that would constitute the beginning of a long and innovative scientific adventure beyond anything he could have ever anticipated. Before one is able to innovate, however, one must acquire both theoretical and practical knowledge, develop critical judgment, and assimilate and rethink the ideas of the day. In 1951, Mirko received his doctorate from the Sorbonne. The same year, he married Monique Lucas, who became his lifetime companion and research assistant.

The early 1950s were times of great advancement and recognition. Like many young scientists of his generation, he questioned the respective roles of RNA and DNA regarding the acquisition of new characteristics (in the case of bacterial resistance).

How could antibiotics communicate with DNA and change its program in order to alter the nucleotide content? What agent selects the choice of amino acids during protein synthesis? DNA? RNA? Enzymes? What are the interactions of these molecules? It was very difficult to conceive, and no one scientist solved this major dilemma. Rather, it was the collective work of hundreds of great minds at laboratories and universities across the globe. Some scientists claimed that it was this or that constituent, others differed. At first, American scientist Oswald Theodore Avery (1877-1955) was strongly criticized for his publication pertaining to cell transformation by DNA. Nobody understood how DNA could select amino acids in order to build peptides (short chains of amino acids) and then proteins. As was everyone else, Mirko was fascinated by all topics pertaining to heredity. He was passionate about the workings of the living world; he thought about it all the time: It was a fantastic challenge for a young biochemist. He always wanted to explore further, which is why, once he finished his doctorate work, Mirko studied organic chemistry, physiology, and embryology.

But then something happened that would change the course of Mirko's life. In 1953, Macheboeuf (who had been injured by chemical gasses during World War I) developed brutal lung cancer. He died that summer. Macheboeuf's death, the completion of his thesis, and his recent marriage drove Mirko to find a more stable position and a lab where he could continue his research.

In France, the Centre National de la Recherche Scientifique (CNRS) financially supports fundamental research with little pressure for a quick return on investment. This gives scientists the leisure to undertake long research without the permanent stress of having to secure funding. The CNRS is a government-funded research organization controlled by the Ministry of Research. Founded in 1939 by governmental decree, the multiple missions of the CNRS include evaluating and carrying out all research capable of advancing scientific knowledge and bringing social, cultural, and economic benefits for society. In 1953, Mirko and his wife, Monique, joined the CNRS and from then on, with grant money, dedicated their efforts and time to fundamental research. Although Mirko could stay at the Pasteur Institute, in the same lab where he had worked on his thesis, Macheboeuf's sudden death had brought about changes in the leadership that didn't agree with Mirko.

CHAPTER TWO

Monod

Jacques Lucien Monod, fine featured, dark, and handsome, with a full head of perfectly coiffed dark hair, was born in Paris on February 9, 1910, to a well-to-do Protestant family. Monod was brilliant, intelligent, and quick. He had been chief of staff of operations for the Forces Françaises de l'Interieur during World War II. In preparation for the Allied landings, he arranged parachute drops of weapons, railroad bombings, and mail interceptions. He was an excellent musician and a highly regarded writer.

Monod obtained his science degree in 1931 and his doctorate in Natural Sciences in 1941. After lecturing at the Faculty of Sciences in 1934 and spending some time at the California Institute of Technology on a Rockefeller grant in 1936, Monod joined the Pasteur Institute as laboratory director under André Lwoff. He was appointed director of the Cell Biochemistry Department in 1954.

"When Monod was elected professor and later made director of our Cell Biochemistry Department, he was very self-centered, bragging about his social connections and boasting about the Rothchild financial support he could receive; he was both efficient and arrogant," Monique recalled during an interview.

As new department head, Monod decided to modernize the old lab and build a brand new lab for cellular biology. During the renovation, the young couple was given the opportunity to spend a few months in the spring of 1953 in Jean Brachet's lab in Belgium. As we have seen already, Brachet was one of the few scientists interested in the role of RNA in the cell.

At that time, the double-helix structure of the DNA had not yet been discovered, nor was the function and existence of RNA known. Today, we have orderly images of DNA, its functioning and of protein synthesis, making it possible for molecular biology to engage in genetic manipulations. The wall prohibiting access to such knowledge back then was still very high.

At the center of our understanding of cancer is DNA, the blueprint of life that holds the plans for our biological fate. DNA was first isolated by the Swiss physician Friedrich Miescher who, in 1869, discovered a microscopic substance in the pus of discarded surgical bandages. As it resided in the nuclei of cells, he called it "nuclein."

Just two years earlier, the Czech monk Gregor Mendel had finished a series of experiments with peas. His observations turned out to be closely connected to the finding of nuclein. Mendel was able to show that certain traits in peas, such as shape or color, were inherited in different packages. These packages are what we now call *genes*.

Yet the connection between genes and nuclein was not clear for many more years. Phoebus Aaron Theodore Levene, M.D., (1869-1940) a biochemist and head of the biochemical laboratory at the Rockefeller Institute of Medical Research in New York, analyzed DNA and found that it contained adenine, guanine, thymine, cytosine, deoxyribose, and a phosphate group. But even Levene, with more than 700 published papers, failed to link genes and inheritance with DNA, as he thought DNA was too simple a chemical molecule.

In 1944, Oswald Theodore Avery succeeded in transferring a hereditary property from one bacterium to another with the aid of pure nucleic acid (DNA). In doing so, he marked the beginning of a new branch of science which has come to be called molecular biology, which, little by little, came to be considered as the basis of genetics.

In 1943, Avery discovered that traits of the "smooth" form of the Pneumococcus could be transferred to the "rough" form of the same bacteria by mixing killed "smooth" bacteria with the live "rough" form.

Avery, along with coworkers Colin MacLeod and Maclyn McCarty, identified DNA as this transforming principle. But this notion was difficult for the scientific community to accept at first.

DNA's role in heredity was confirmed in 1953, when Alfred Hershey and Martha Chase, in the now famous Hershey-Chase experiment, showed that DNA is the genetic material of the famously physiologically simple T2 bacteriophage. A *bacteriophage* (from *bacteria* and the Greek *phagein*, "to eat") is any one of a number of viruses that infect bacteria. The term is commonly used in its shortened form, *phage*.

In 1953, based on X-ray diffraction images taken by Rosalind Franklin at King's College and the information that the bases were paired, James D. Watson and Francis Crick suggested what is now accepted as the first accurate model of the DNA structure in the journal *Nature*.

As the *Time 100* (*Time* magazine's 100 most important people of the century) scientist and thinkers category notes, "On Feb. 28, 1953, Francis Crick walked into the Eagle Pub in Cambridge, England, and, as James Watson later recalled, announced that 'we have found the secret of life.' Actually, they had. That morning, Watson and Crick had figured out the structure of deoxyribonucleic acid, DNA. And that structure—a 'double helix' that can 'unzip' to make copies of itself—confirmed suspicions that DNA carries life's hereditary information."

Although Watson and Crick won the Nobel Prize in Physiology or Medicine in 1962, they were strongly indebted to Franklin at King's College who was creating the world's best X-ray diffraction pictures of DNA. She provided the experimental evidence for Watson and Crick's model as part of a series of five articles in the same issue of *Nature*. However, speculation continues on who should have received credit for the discovery, as it was based on Franklin's data—and she was also working toward the final interpretation of DNA, that it was able to divide, and when healthy, make perfect complementary matches. Tragically, Franklin died of cancer in 1958 at 37, never receiving the credit that she so deserved.

These findings represent the birth of molecular biology and genetics and the fountainhead of the river down which modern molecular scientists travel.

The publication by Watson and Crick on April 25, 1953, in *Nature* created a shock in the scientific world: The double-helix model discovered by the authors was a true revolution in the field of molecular biology. Two months later the same authors published a new article describing the sequence of the A, G, T, C bases that carry the genetic information. If we compare a nucleic acid with language, we can think of the building blocks as the letters of the alphabet. With this analogy, we may say that the language of nucleic acids describes our main inherited or genetic traits. It tells us if our eyes and those of our children are blue or brown; if we are tall or short.

From then on, DNA and genes became paramount and marked the development of a molecular biology focused entirely on genetics. Genes determined the line up of amino acids in the proteins. The double-helix model was a beautiful and elegant scientific achievement. Mirko bowed to this success without any bitterness and told Monique: "They did a better job than we did."

Yet the idea that changes to the three-dimensional structure of the DNA play a central role in cancer was ignored in favor of identifying the actual sequences of the building blocks of the DNA (adenine, cytosine, guanine and thymine) and changes in this genetic sequence (mutations). Virtually the entire scientific world now looked at a three-dimensional world as if it were linear and flat.

Today, we know that DNA is a nucleic acid that contains the genetic instructions used in the development and functioning of all known living organisms. The main role of DNA molecules is the long-term storage of information, and DNA is often likened to a set of blueprints, etched in stone, that contains the instructions needed to construct other components of cells, such as RNA molecules and proteins. The DNA segments that carry this genetic information are called genes, but other DNA sequences have structural purposes or are involved in regulating genetic information. "Your DNA is your fate" is a simple way of summing up many scientists' views in the past 40 years on DNA. Little did they credit environmental cross-talk as the most significant influence on one's DNA. It was a tragic mistake in thinking—one that played so well into the hands of industrial interests. The greatest proponent in France of omnipotent DNA would prove to be Monod.

Chemically, DNA is a long polymer of simple units called nucleotides, with a backbone made of sugars and phosphate groups joined by ester bonds. Attached to each sugar is one of four types of molecules called bases. It is the sequence of these four bases along the backbone that encodes information. This information is read using the genetic code, which specifies the sequence of the amino acids within proteins. The code is read by copying stretches of DNA into the related messenger nucleic acid RNA, in a process called *transcription*. The messenger RNA molecules are necessary to synthesize proteins, but other RNAs are used directly in structures such as ribosomes and spliceosomes.

Within cells, DNA is organized into structures called chromosomes and the set of chromosomes within a cell make up a genome. These chromosomes are duplicated before cells divide, in a process called DNA replication. Eukaryotic organisms such as animals, plants, and fungi store their DNA inside the cell nucleus, while in prokaryotes such as bacteria it is found in the cell's cytoplasm. Within the chromosomes, chromatin proteins such as histones compact and organize DNA to control its interactions with other proteins as well as which genes are transcribed.

The concept that DNA contains genetic information—specific sequences of nucleotides that code for specific proteins—has had a far greater impact on cancer research than the idea that DNA exists as a fully three-dimensional double-helical structure. Monod, Beljanski's chief opponent, accepted and passionately defended the absolute supremacy of DNA in genetics. Yet in his own writings, Beljanski observed, "In those years, one had just assimilated the new biology concepts borne of Watson and Crick's discoveries concerning the genetic code." What he had come up with he said, "was a beautiful new vision of how the program of each living cell is registered in a long molecule in the form of a double helix: the DNA. It is the basis of all life forms, the genealogy book of the human species if you will. But in the years following this fundamental discovery and the excitement of finally understanding the genetic code, many researchers came to believe that unraveling the code would explain the evolution of life and the appearance of most, if not all, pathologies. For them, there was no alternative to the supremacy of genes, no possible modulation of that program. Soon, and particularly in France, it became an imposed dogma (the central dogma) without any possible alternative." Still today, "you must pretend that you are a neodarwinian (evolution = genes + selection) whatever your ideas are in reality, otherwise you are socially and scientifically dead" (as in Jean Staune's "Notre existence a-t-elle un sens?" *Presse de la Renaissance*, Paris 2007).

Thus, the geneticists in France, such as Monod, dominated modern medical French research. Mirko, like many other biochemists, was trying to figure out the still unknown mechanism of protein synthesis, whose connection with RNA was not suspected.

After Machebœuf died and their time working with Brachet had elapsed, the renovation work of the lab at the Pasteur Institute was not over, and Severo Ochoa of New York University invited the young couple to join his laboratory. "It was major," recalls Monique. "We were overjoyed to go to America. The research was cutting edge."

In 1954, Severo Ochoa had been appointed chairman of the Department of Biochemistry at New York University. Indeed, Ochoa and his team had just discovered an enzyme, polyribonucleotide phosphorylase (PNPase), which was capable of producing the *in vitro* synthesis of small RNAs.

Ochoa was aware that Mirko had been publishing papers on the accumulation of RNA in resistant bacteria. Knowing about his work, Ochoa invited the

Beljanskis to New York on a two-year scholarship. At that time, Monique was pregnant with their first child, Sylvie.

Entry into the United States was complicated by the fact that Mirko was still a Yugoslav national. At the height of the McCarthy era, this posed problems in terms of obtaining an entry visa. The Democratic Federal Yugoslavia had been proclaimed in 1943 by Yugoslav partisans who fought in the resistance movement in World War II. In 1946, a socialist government was established and the nation was renamed the Federal People's Republic of Yugoslavia.

Monod set up a meeting for Mirko with his friend, the vice-consul of the United States Embassy. During the meeting, they talked about Yugoslavian politics. Suddenly, according to Monique, "He asked Mirko to take certain political stances against Yugoslavia in order to acquire his U.S. visa." Mirko refused outright and abruptly left. We can ask ourselves whether or not it was Monod who suggested such a bargain in order to "test" Mirko to see whether he was "buyable." When Mirko returned to the Pasteur Institute, Monod was eating lunch at the grand table, surrounded by his collaborators. Monique recalled their interaction:

"So Mirko, it went well?"

"No!" Mirko furiously recounted the interview in front of everyone.

Monod flushed and responded dryly, "You must have misunderstood."

"No, no, I have understood very well, and it's scandalous!"

The couple abandoned the idea of going to the United States. Monod avoided them when they entered Pasteur's grounds; a heavy malaise was very perceptible. They returned to their work.

A few weeks later, Monique decided to release some steam; she grabbed the telephone and impetuously and rather brutally told the United States Consulate that they were going to publish in the press the content of the propositions made by the vice-consul. Then, calmly, with great relief, she went back to work and forgot about it. Two days later, Mirko's visa for the United States arrived…on the desk of Monod. He handed Mirko the document without a word.

MOVING FORWARD

The research Mirko performed with Ochoa in New York resulted in three papers published by the duo in 1958, a year before Ochoa would win the Nobel Prize. With Arthur Kornberg, Ochoa received the 1959 Nobel Prize in Physiology or Medicine for their discovery of the mechanisms in the biological synthesis of

RNA. Knowing that all life stems from the interactions of proteins and nucleic acids and because the genetic code was not yet established, the famous biochemist's papers with Beljanski were important to advancing understanding of how RNA plays an important intermediate role in protein synthesis. For only a few years, scientists had suspected the relationship between proteins and RNA but had yet to discover the details.

In as much as nucleic acids and proteins were thought to be the two main principles of life, it seemed highly probable that the proteins should take part in the rebuilding of nucleic acids. Proteins, in the form of enzymes, take part in practically every chemical reaction in the biological world. If DNA dictates orders for protein synthesis via messenger RNA, DNA must then be synthesized of and by proteins! It is to the everlasting credit of Ochoa to have uncovered this fundamental mechanism by which a special type of enzyme can build up RNA in test tubes without any template.

In those days in New York, both Beljanski and Ochoa showed that small RNAs indeed play a role in the synthesis of proteins, since they could demonstrate a certain specificity of binding between a given RNA polymer and a given amino acid.

Yet, Ochoa never realized RNA was interacting with both the micro and macro environments of the body and the world—and that RNA could dictate to DNA. DNA, thanks to the dogmas of Watson and Crick, reigned as the omnipotent master of our biological fate.

Yet if he did not succeed in winning the genetic-code race, Mirko learned much during his research, in particular, the importance of different RNAs in the process of cell duplication and transcription. His intellectual independence kept him aloof from the fashionable interpretations of his time, the rigid dogma postulating the omnipotent role of DNA, while assigning to messenger RNA the unique role of intermediary between DNA and proteins. Despite the fact that Ochoa graciously proposed that Mirko stay in the United States, Mirko felt he owed a debt to France. Burning with a passion to take his RNA research further, Mirko returned to France.

CHAPTER THREE

Homecoming

In the spring of 1959, Mirko and Monique returned to France to work in Monod's department. With Monique's parents altogether joyous to look after their baby Sylvie, Mirko and Monique agreed they would work long hours in the lab to pursue their research. By now, however, Monod had been appointed director of the Pasteur Institute, and his grip on power had become absolute.

In his rise to power, Monod had purged the Pasteur Institute of all dissenters, and there were many. He was not well-liked initially, as the purge occurred. He was able to very quickly eliminate any opposition from former directors and professors such as Jacques Tréfoul, a former head of the Pasteur Institute who had discovered the first bactericide sulfamid. Professor Pierre Lépine, head of the virology department and "father" of the first oral polio vaccine, was also marginalized, as were many others.

Monique claims, "He went as far as firing several scientists who were close to retirement; in so doing, he humiliated them, and as a result, everyone feared him. He became increasingly authoritarian and rigid."

Mirko informed Monod that he wished to go on with his studies pertaining to the *in vitro* synthesis of peptides (very short stretches of proteins) in the presence of a variety of RNA compounds.

Monod responded, "But the whole world works on *my* ideas!"

Quietly, Mirko answered, "That makes a lot of people; all the more reason to give me liberty!"

In fact, everything was different between them. Monod never performed any experiments himself. While his staff did the experiments, Monod did the synthesis thereafter. On the other hand, Mirko loved to do experiments, making his own controls and constructing his hypotheses step by step. He would stay in the lab

10 hours per day in front of his test tubes without speaking. He worked like this for more than 50 years. He never tired and was literally obsessed with his work. Mirko was very demanding of himself and of the people working with him.

With the rise of genetics, Monod adhered more and more to the dogma of an omnipotent DNA, complete with set roles for each cog in the mechanics of gene regulation and expression, which could be accomplished exclusively through intermediary proteins with the help of messenger and transfer RNAs. In so doing, he was also promoting his own work and finding the support of the wider global scientific community.

But now, if he did not have the whole world working on his ideas, he certainly had many of the best minds of the Pasteur Institute doing so. With André Lwoff and François Jacob, the three formed a domineering and cohesive team (all the more once they shared the Nobel Prize)—and, of course, these men recognized early on that their Nobel fortunes were tied together.

Lwoff (1902–1994) was the French microbiologist who in 1925 began a long association with the Pasteur Institute. In the 1920s he studied morphogenesis—the growth and differentiation of form and structure in an organism. In particular, he investigated one-celled protozoans, which led to the discovery of the transmission of genes that occur outside the nucleus (*extranuclear inheritance*) in these organisms. His treatise *L'Évolution Pysiologique*, published in 1941, developed the thesis of biochemical evolution by progressive losses of biosynthetic capacity and accounted for the rise of parasitism, since as an organism loses its biosynthetic capacity, it must (almost out of necessity) take on such a role. He shared the 1965 Nobel Prize in Physiology or Medicine with Monod and Jacob for his discovery that the genetic material of a virus can be assimilated by bacteria and passed on to succeeding generations. Jacob joined the Pasteur Institute under Dr. Lwoff in 1950. He was appointed laboratory director in 1956, and then in 1960 led the recently created Department of Cell Genetics.

Crick's central dogma was that information flow was from DNA to RNA via the process of transcription, the making of a single-stranded RNA molecule off a DNA template. Messenger RNA used translation, which is the construction of an amino acid sequence (polypeptide), to combine these to make even more variant, perhaps endless, proteins. But the rigid program originated with DNA.

In 1960, Monod and Jacob isolated messenger RNA, the information vector between the DNA of the nucleus and the cytoplasmic ribosome where proteins are synthesized. This put them in the ballgame for a Nobel Prize. The discovery marked the apex of the "central dogma of molecular biology" as stated by Crick, which declares that the gene is at the center of all biological reactions, and therefore sanctifies genetic determinism. From then on, no one could escape this dogma…and certainly not a scientist at the Pasteur Institute—certainly not Mirko.

The primacy of DNA was absolute—particularly by 1965 when the trio shared the Nobel Prize.

DNA FLOW

As a consequence of the DNA dogma, the constant litany of the molecular biologists was the promise of genetic research curing every illness. It was a scientific gravy train because it would involve a seemingly endless need for research—much valued research. Research funds were being granted by the federal National Institutes of Health and institutions throughout Europe, but only for those scientists in line with the new genetics.

Because of state and industry interests and their close alliance throughout the world, strategic choices of research were decided in the interest of the profits of the chemical and pharmaceutical industries, which often had nothing to do with humanity's immediate needs for curing or palliating disease.

The excess and frenzy toward genetics was not without serious repercussions. In the 19th century, it was used as a cover for racist persecutions led by civilized nations such as Australia, America, and Africa. It helped give rise to eugenics, and in the 20th century, Nazism channeled biological research and funding into genetics.

If the deciphering of the genome was to become the holy grail of future therapies, it was necessary to keep investors on their toes (banks, donors, public funds…), in favor of genetics, as well as to justify the claims that new treatments were coming and new genetic tests were being constantly developed. Stocks rose, patents were filed, and licenses sold, thanks to the new market for genetic research and potential applications…it became the business of science!

CHAPTER FOUR

New King

Monod won the Nobel Prize in 1965 together with Lwoff and Jacob for explaining how messenger and transfer RNA (tRNA) took direction from DNA to create an endless number of amino acids that would lead to peptides and longer stranded proteins. At the height of his Nobel success, however, the walls around him were crumbling, and he had so little time left himself.

Mirko kept on the trail of other types of RNA, ignoring Monod who ordered all at Pasteur to work solely on the central dogma and accept the "messenger boy" status of RNA. Not that Monod himself hadn't turned his attention to RNA; indeed, he had as well, but he was attempting to subjugate the importance of RNA—as much as he desired to suppress the intellect and findings of Mirko.

One of Mirko's favorite authors at the time was the Austrian Stefan Zweig, a writer of the early 20th century who authored *Erasmus of Rotterdam*. Erasmus, born in 1466 or 1469, was not afraid to criticize contemporary Christian beliefs and wrote satirical attacks on the traditions of the Catholic Church and popular superstitions, such as *The Praise of Folly*, which he dedicated to Sir Thomas Moore. Moore was beheaded in 1535 when he refused to sign the Act of Supremacy that declared Henry VIII Supreme Head of the Church in England. One quote from the book perfectly illustrates Mirko's viewpoint regarding science: "Man in all its humanity has the duty not to conform but to fight the enemy of free thinking and to remain truthful to his own ideal as opposed to his clan." As he had left Serbia, so had he left orthodoxy at Pasteur.

Mirko was on a path that was far out of line with the glory seekers or even of his own clan, for he had no plans for fame. He was a foreigner at a sophisticated and powerful institution. Throughout the late '50s and early '60s, he continued to work his own way, quietly in his laboratory. In keeping with his interest in plants, Mirko decided to look into the mechanisms through which the soil bacteria, *Agrobacterium tumefaciens*, induces cancerous tumors in plants (called *Crown gall*). Like several other scientists, he thought that RNA could be an oncogenic agent. His friend, Maurice Stroun, had recently shown this in a 1971 article in the *Journal of Bacteriology* (106;2;634-9) and Mirko wanted to directly isolate the RNA and demonstrate its ability to induce plant cancer disease. He teamed up with plant oncologists from the department at the Pasteur Institute to better understand the mechanisms by which the bacteria induce the cell transformation into cancer. This was highly unusual in Monod's lab. They succeeded and published in the *Proceeding of the National Academy of Science* their discovery of the oncogenic RNA that the bacteria injects into the plant in order to induce the cancer called Crown Gall. In other words, it was a demonstration that this type of RNA may, by itself, trigger the behavior of DNA.

Mirko also returned to his earlier work on antibiotic resistance and studied bacterial resistance to showdomycin. This antibiotic, extracted from a microscopic mushroom (*showdoensis*) from the Far East, is a natural nucleotide, almost pure nucleic acid; a simple, beautiful model. Its structure is very similar to that of uridine, a component of RNA. Because of this resemblance, Mirko hoped it would have an effect on the nucleic acid of the bacteria.

For Mirko, this simple model was the beginning of numerous critical discoveries concerning the impact of biological or chemical agents on the functioning of DNA and environmentally induced cancers. They showed that RNA, as well as many environmental influences, trigger gene expression.

All bacteria became resistant to showdomycin in his experiments and had two times more purine bases (G and A) in their RNA compared to wild-type nonresistant bacteria, but Mirko and Monique noted that the base content of their DNA was not modified—even though they now could survive the effects of the antibiotics. This implied that the RNA was not coded by the DNA—but what's more, the RNA was making basic changes to the bacterial form that led to its quick adaptation to the antibiotic.

In addition, they observed that the resistant bacteria excrete a "transformant RNA." This, in turn, is able to modify *Escherichia coli* bacteria and transform other types of bacteria, as well.[3,4,5]

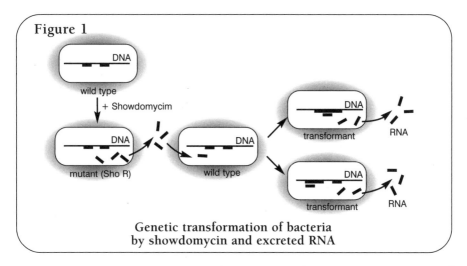

**Genetic transformation of bacteria
by showdomycin and excreted RNA**

The team then showed (see Figure 1) that the "transformant RNA" is synthesized in the bacteria by polynucleotide phosphoryase (the Ochoa enzyme on which both scientists worked a few years earlier), independently of a DNA template. It normally remained inactive in wild-type bacteria. Under the proper conditions, however, Mirko found it would become activated and use a short transformant RNA as a template. This is what happens in transformants under the influence of the antibiotic showdomycin. This mechanism certainly plays an essential role during the acquisition of resistance of both bacteria and cells and probably played a role in evolution. Dr. Bonissol, from the Viral Department at the Pasteur Institute, confirmed this strange phenomenon on human cells in cultures in the presence of showdomycin.

The transforming RNA has another job to perform: It can bring information to bacteria and also modify bacteria of a species other than the one from which it was created. The transformed strains contained no trace of the transformant RNA and therefore had transferred and assimilated seamlessly information from one bacterial strain to another! It was the proof that RNA (a nonmutagenic element) can cause a stable, hereditary transformation. The possibility of transforming bacteria by means of DNA had been known for a long time, since Avery's work on Pneumococcus appeared in 1944. (Avery also had a difficult time having his work recognized and accepted.)

Now for the first time in the history of biology, proof existed that RNA, until then relegated to the role of subordinate tasks such as a mere intermediary between DNA and proteins, can transmit information and determine cellular fate, as does DNA. But what was the mechanism of such events?

Mirko's results would change the vision of science—and now he had to do battle with Monod. He did not know then, not yet, how it would be seen decades later. He never would.

Without rejecting the prevalent scientific ideas (DNA→mRNA→Proteins), Mirko by now thought that many other factors were also very important to the cell: particularly environmental trigger molecules including peptides, hormones, pesticides, antibiotics, pollutants, and, of course, as he now knew, various RNAs....

How could an "excreted RNA" be a vector of information and transform bacteria in a permanent state?

Nothing in nature is useless, especially not an enzyme. Mirko postulated the existence of an enzyme in bacteria that could transfer information from RNA into DNA. One may imagine that such an enzyme would be a thorn in the side of the central dogma, and it enraged Monod.

But the walls surrounding Monod's work were crumbling elsewhere, too. Just a few months before in the United States, during the first half of the decade of the 1970s, Dr. Howard M. Temin of the McArdle Laboratory, University of Wisconsin, discovered an enzyme in an RNA virus that was able to copy RNA into DNA. This was exactly the reverse of the transcription of DNA into RNA, the only accepted possibility until then. The enzyme responsible was called *reverse transcriptase*, and the virus using this enzyme to multiply in the cell was called a *retrovirus*. However, Temin's discovery pertained only to viral biology, already an unorthodox field in regard to bacterial cellular biology. And even then, Temin encountered difficulties in getting his results recognized.

Temin's description of how tumor viruses act on the genetic material of the cell through reverse transcription was revolutionary for its day. This upset the widely held belief at the time of the "central dogma" of molecular biology that believed genetic information to flow exclusively from DNA to RNA to protein. Temin showed that certain tumor viruses carried the enzymatic ability to reverse the flow of information from RNA back to DNA using reverse transcriptase. This phenomenon was also independently and simultaneously discovered by David Baltimore, with whom Temin shared the Nobel Prize.

In 1971, only a few months after Temin's work was published, Beljanski became the first to show that reverse transcriptase indeed existed in bacteria. Indeed, Mirko was first with this very relevant finding (since bacteria are considered to closely mirror a simplified version of human genetics), and in 1989 in the

December 7 issue of the journal *Nature* (342:624) Temin acknowledged in a retrocitation that Beljanski was the first to discover in bacteria what we now know of now as reverse transcriptase. His retrocitation included the following four seminal published studies:

- Beljanski, M. C. r. hebd. Seanc. Acad. Sci., Paris D274, 2801–2804 (1972).
- Buljanski, M. C. r. hebd. Séanc. Acad. Sci., Paris D276, 1625–1628 (1973).
- Beljanski, M. & Beljanski, M. Biochem. Genet. 17, 163–180 (1974).
- Beljanski, M., Bourgarel, P. & Beljanski, M.S. C. r. hebd. Sesnc. Acad. Sci., Paris D286. 1825–1828 (1978).

Monod knew that such results would be a damaging blow to the existing dogma by definitively showing RNA, like DNA, could not only contain but also transmit genetic information. Mirko's research had opened up new perspectives in biology, in the process of evolution, and oncogenesis.

Monod was absolutely furious: He considered these results to clash with the supreme notion of DNA. Monod was all the more upset because in his just-published book, *Chance and Necessity*, he claimed that "It has never been observed and is not even conceivable that information could move from the reverse direction."

Although Temin was working on a viral replication process that was not considered to be relevant to bacterial forms, when Mirko showed Monod in his own lab that reverse transcriptase also existed in bacteria, Monod barked, "You will not publish these results!"

"What a reckless statement!" Mirko told Monod.

Matured and hardened by years of research and observation, Mirko disregarded Monod's prohibition against publishing his results, and some five articles appeared in 1972 and 1973.[6,7,8,9,10]

Professor P. P. Grassé, a renowned comparative zoologist, wrote in his book *L'Evolution du Vivant* (Les Editions Albin Michel, 1973), "The ink of Monod's lines had not even dried when he was given a fierce denial with no chance for appeal. The logic of living things was not Monod's logic, but nature's logic. The beautiful structure showed cracks."

An important aspect of cellular biology had been unlocked, thanks to these findings. Reverse transcriptase is now a "star" enzyme. Incorporation of foreign RNA into a genome is now considered a common occurrence, observed in viruses, microorganisms, plants and animals. In the human genome, the presence of certain sequences of DNA reflects the transcription of short RNA of diverse origins.

In brief, the latter has been transcribed into DNA. For example, reverse transcriptase from an animal cell can transcribe RNA of viral origin into DNA.

The discovery of reverse transcriptase is one of the most important of the modern era of medicine, as reverse transcriptase is the central enzyme in several widespread human diseases, such as HIV, the virus that causes AIDS, and hepatitis B.

Monod was getting sick. He had cancer. He was dying. Monique recounted their last meeting which took place in March 1976 at 10 in the morning in the large office of the director of the Pasteur Institute in Paris, in the presence of Joel de Rosnay (Director of Development) and Christiane Bonissol, Ph.D., head of the Virology lab at the Pasteur Institute.

Mirko and Monique clearly saw that their boss was sickened, probably with cancer, and he acknowledged that illness with a reference to the hope that the genetic system would lead to a cure. But the two men argued and Mirko accused Monod of attempting to suppress his work.

All traditional cancer treatments are quite aggressive and compromise or destroy patients' immunity, leaving them susceptible to many types of infection. More and more concerned with problems of oncogenesis, Mirko felt the pressure of humanity. Where was all of this research pointed if not toward the benefit of the people? His association with Ochoa was also now paying off.

During this time, Mirko worked like a master molecular biologist: under normal conditions, at 70 degrees centigrade, and providing the Ochoa enzyme with the four different nucleotides (A, G, C, U) that make up RNA, he synthesized *in vitro* an RNA molecule. Then by cutting the ribopolymer forming at the C and U bases, which it cleaved at that temperature, the final molecule favored the accumulation of A and G bases. Under the conditions of the experiment, the PNPase (a thermo-resistant enzyme) was protected to a certain degree by the presence of magnesium ions and the substrates on which it acted, and it performed admirably at this high temperature. In this way, Beljanski and his colleagues succeeded in synthesizing in the test tube a small RNA in which the ratio between the purine and pyrimidine bases was close to 2:1. They would now test this activity in the synthesis of DNA.[11]

A highly purified bone marrow DNA as template, *without any trace of RNA*, was introduced into a mixture containing all the preliminary matter needed for the synthesis of DNA (the four deoxyribonucleotides, buffer, magnesium, and a polymerization enzyme called *DNA-dependent DNA polymerase* because it synthesizes DNA from a template DNA). Why would he pick bone marrow to start with?

Because that's what chemotherapy and radiation therapy attacked. *But nothing happened.* Without a catalyst, the DNA was relatively impotent to do much of anything. It needed something. It needed RNA.

Then the researchers added the newly synthesized RNA, and the replication of DNA was stimulated in a spectacular way, as shown in Figure 2.

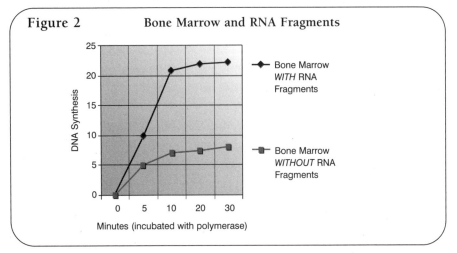

Figure 2   Bone Marrow and RNA Fragments

Its synthesis was stimulated by the small RNA, rich in purine bases. There was no other intervention of the RNA primer except to initiate replication, which was carried out normally. Once the priming work was completed, the small RNA primer is released and eliminated by the nucleases that are always present.

Now the team worked feverishly to develop a preparation. They had something that could aid in the amplification of DNA synthesis. Yet the process of *in vitro* enzymatic synthesis of primer RNA was long, costly, and provided very little material. To pursue the research regarding the primers and produce them in large quantities, Mirko got the idea to prepare RNA fragments. It was simple and the material was easy to purify. Mirko worked with long bacterial chains of RNA that were isolated, highly purified and cut in different fragments depending on the choice of the ribonuclease and experimental conditions. In order to stay as close as possible to natural and physiological conditions, Mirko chose bacteria of the human intestinal tract as a source of RNA and enzymatically cut the long bacterial RNA into fragments. (It would require some 10 years of arduous work to pass all the tests and be able to produce safe, selective, specific primers for bone marrow DNA.) In the course of their work, they found other primers, specific to other applications (bacteriophages and others which deserved follow-up and new scientists to take their work further), but they focused on the RNA primer specifically active with bone marrow DNA.

Bone marrow stem cells are the locus for the formation of immune cells (i.e., white blood cells and platelets), but chemotherapy destroys them in patients. Patients have to stop their rounds to allow their bodies to recover, thus making the treatment less effective. But what if the bone marrow cells could be protected and the patient could go through all their rounds and their survival could be enhanced?

In vitro, these RNA fragments were used as primers to initiate the replication of DNA(s) isolated from rabbit bone marrow and spleen; they are inactive with DNA isolated from several other normal tissues and cancerous cells, including cancerous bone marrow cells.

In order to control whether the production of bone marrow DNA provided more stem cells and led to an increase of immune cells, the team had to proceed with biological models. But the Institute denied them access to the animal husbandry. However, a colleague secretly gave them access to his own husbandry where they kept a few rabbits that they first exposed to chemotherapy drugs (CP) in order to destroy their immune system, as is the case in humans during cancer treatments.

In the evening, a member of the Beljanski team drew blood samples which he quickly took to an outside medical lab. Every other day he had to verify the status of the rabbits' white blood cells and platelets. Work in such conditions was slow, but the scientists' determination remained undeterred.

In experimental rabbits, a few doses of RNA fragments restored, in a rapid and harmless way, normal genesis of leukocyte and platelet levels when these had been drastically decreased by the CPs.

In addition, an imbalance between polynuclear and lymphocyte count provoked in rabbits by several drugs used in chemotherapy was rapidly corrected by treating the animal with active RNA fragments.

Granulocyte/lymphocyte balance, upset by daily CP administration, was also restored during the increase of both types of cells. No toxicity was observed, and numerous repeated doses of RNA fragments showed no cumulative effect and did not lead to a loss of leukopoietic-stimulating activity.

Tumor-bearing rabbits and mice could also be protected using RNA fragments against the toxic effect of CP without impeding the anticancer activity of this drug (see Figure 3).

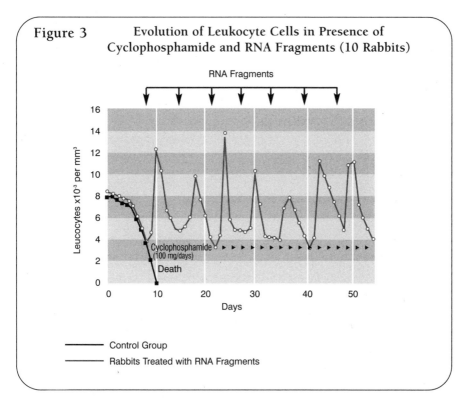

Figure 3 — Evolution of Leukocyte Cells in Presence of Cyclophosphamide and RNA Fragments (10 Rabbits)

Beljanski termed these new molecules "primers." The French team was the first one to achieve the synthesis and/or manufacture of RNAs active in the replication of DNA. Monod died in 1976 and was buried in Cannes on the French Riviera. Indeed, the hostility and cold lack of interest shown by the Pasteur Institute in the RNA fragments' ability to boost immunity led Mirko to contact the Mérieux Institute, a large French pharmaceutical group with a good reputation and a relative interest in natural substances. The Mérieux Institute was located a few miles north of Lyons in the Rhône Valley.

Management there took an immediate interest in the RNA fragments. At the time, the only treatment available was blood transfusions to protect patients from the drop in white blood cell counts (aplasia) and/or platelets (thrombocytopenia). Those were the days of the infamous blood contamination scandal that killed many AIDS and hepatitis patients in France.

The Mérieux Institute immediately signed a contract for the production of Beljanski RNA fragments. Everything was going well. Charles Mérieux, CEO of Mérieux Institute, sent the CNRS a letter confirming the product's efficacy in animals receiving a high dosage of chemotherapy. But even with this backing, the Pasteur Institute and the CNRS remained hostile and never improved Mirko's working conditions.

Mérieux Institute
17 rue Bourgelat
69002
Lyons

October 6, 1976

Mr. Berkaloff, Director of CNRS
National Center for Scientific Research
Paris

Dear Mr. Director,

I would like to bring to your attention the fact that, in our research departments, we have reproduced the results reported by Dr. Beljanski, head of research at C.N.R.S. (cellular biology), concerning his product "RLB."

Dr. Beljanski has, in effect, entrusted us with samples of his product "RLB." In our hands, an injection allowed for the restoration of normal rates of leukocytes in animals who are severely and consistently immunodepressed, whether by Cyclophosphamide or Methotrexate.

Sincerely yours, Charles Mérieux

For four years, the Mérieux Institute continued to study and produce RNA fragments. They were very pleased with them, offered them to numerous doctors, and Mérieux himself proclaimed his satisfaction everywhere.

Yet even with such important results, more trouble was to be heaped upon Mirko.

His results were announced in the Académie des Sciences, February 9, 1977, by the renowned virologist and polio vaccine researcher Pierre Lépine, the head of the Department of Virology at Pasteur, who was not afraid to highlight, on such an occasion, the new importance of RNA primers. In this case, RNA primers only initiated the replication of DNA and did not interfere with its quality (primers are never integrated into the DNA). Indeed, in so doing, Lépine challenged Monod's central dogma, and, in supporting Beljanski, he embarassed Monod. Then suddenly, the relationship with Mérieux soured: The Mérieux Institute merged with the Pasteur Institute. The new entity, called Pasteur-Mérieux, became the number-one lab for vaccines in France. In this context, Mérieux's relationship with Mirko crumbled. The contract was abruptly cancelled without any honest and decent justification. "For the next few years, the management of the Pasteur Institute had relegated us to two rooms (with a cold chamber) in the basement," recalled Monique of this period in the mid to late '70s. "The newer equipment (centrifuges, radioactivity counters…) were found on the upper floor, but some older machines that were still perfectly functional were left in the basement, not far from us. In order not to be inconvenienced, we took up the habit of using the machines in the basement as much as possible, which, in effect, we were the only ones to use."

After the death of Monod, J. P. Aubert had been named director of the Department of Biochemistry and Microbial Genetics, formerly the Department of Biochemistry, the department where Mirko had worked since his entry into the Pasteur Institute in 1948. When Mirko refused to stop publishing and, indeed, enlisted support from prestigious scientists associated with Pasteur, this proved too much, too threatening. Their continued research, conducted enthusiastically and producing results, annoyed Aubert. He sent Mirko and Monique a letter on January 11, 1978, prohibiting them from continuing their work in any capacity in his department. The Institute had established an irrevocable commitment to not only ostracizing and shunning them, but now, banning them.

At the receipt of J. P. Aubert's letter, while they tried to find a solution, they had experiments to finish; in particular, they had to go to the radioactivity counter and read the results of their last experiment. But a trap was waiting for them: the vice-director of the Institute (a work colleague) had stationed two people behind a door, waiting for either Mirko or Monique to come and use the counter. "When Mirko appeared, a man vigorously objected to his using the counter. Mirko returned, white with rage. Monique tried to calm him and said, 'I will go a little later, when he has left.'"

One or two hours later she went with the little radioactive vials on a tray; the man was still there, waiting to confront her and said, "You do not have the right to pass!"

January 11, 1978

Dear Colleague,

Following the letter D/77-5-n 655 from the Director of the Pasteur Institutes, from the 20th of December 1977, the Council of Biochemistry and Genetic Microbiology examined, in the meeting on January 10, 1978, the new situation that results in the General Director's decision to cancel the credit and personnel for the BGM department granted in 1977, in compensation for the availability of working conditions that the Department has provided for you. [The real purpose was to stop the funding that the Beljanski team needed to continue its work.]

Faced with the decision of the Director, the Council of the Department came to the conclusion that the Department was not able to continue to provide your group with the material support that you have benefited from until now. Consequentially, I regret to inform you that as of January 1978:

1. You will not have access to the local services of the Department: heat rooms, cold rooms, black rooms, libraries or kitchens.

2. You will no longer benefit from any help within the Department regardless of the type of work at hand.

3. You may no longer use the Department's equipment, in particular: dishwashers, autoclaves, centrifuges, radiation gauges, spectrophotometers or copy machines.

4. You may no longer use the basic supply of products provided by the Department, in particular, chemical products, cultures or glassware.

Sincerely yours, J. P. Aubert
Head of the Department of Biochemistry and Microbiology

She told him that this was ridiculous and tried to go around him. "So, he pushed me, caught me by the hair and threw me to the ground. I am not very big and I had my hands full, so I could not defend myself! Furious, I insulted him."

At this moment, his two accomplices came out from hiding behind the door and he exclaimed, "You heard, she insulted me!"

Monique returned to their small laboratory where, less than an hour later, a letter came "to us to tell us that I had one hour to leave the Institute where I had worked for 23 years. Mirko had just until the end of the month to clear the laboratory of our personal effects. In the meantime, we knew that a warning had been sent out to the different laboratories and institutes of Paris not to give us accommodation."

On March 17, 1978, F. Gros, general director of the Pasteur Institute, wrote another letter dictating that they must leave the premises immediately to never return.

Mr. Beljanski,

Following the incident that occurred yesterday between yourself and Mrs. Beljanski on one side and Ferreira and Goldberg on the other side, and after Mr. Virat had heard the versions of the events presented by Mrs. Beljanski [in reality he refused to listen to her] and Mr. Goldberg, I have made the following decisions:

Access to the Pasteur Institute is, as of this evening, March 17, 1978 at 6 o'clock, strictly forbidden to Mrs. Monique Beljanski.

Use of the laboratory granted to you by the direction of the Pasteur Institute will be henceforth prohibited to you, and you must vacate the premises by noon on March 30th at the latest.

All fundamental research activity will be forbidden to you as of this date on the premises of the Pasteur Institute until further notice.

F. Gros, General Director

In 1978, Mirko and Monique left Pasteur. It was all over.

CHAPTER FIVE

Radiation Protection

Against the Pasteur Institute's will, the small team found a home at the University of Châtenay Malabry School of Pharmacy (which is part of the Université Paris-Sud), located about 12 miles from Paris. They were offered two large rooms, empty of any type of equipment but with access to animal husbandry. They received no funding from the CNRS or from the university, but Mirko won an important contract with the research services of the French Army to work on radioprotection. Human skin scarring, known as fibrosis, is caused by radiotherapy. The same type of radiation damage was also being noted by the military among its personnel as a result of the use of nuclear energy. Landing the research contract was certainly financially fortunate but fortuitous also because, on top of the research requested by the Army, they could pursue and deepen their own research with the RNA fragments and a special extract of the *Ginkgo biloba* tree. While this research was somewhat tangential to Mirko's more fundamental discoveries, from the unique perspective and needs of the cancer patient and oncologist, it is nonetheless quite important and provides a complement to his later discovery of destabilized DNA.

The *Ginkgo biloba* tree is believed to be over 270 million years old. Individual trees may live as long as 1,000 years, growing to a height of 100 to 122 feet and with a trunk diameter of 3 to 4 feet. The tree is originally native to China and Japan, but has since been extensively cultivated throughout the world, due to its hardy nature. *Ginkgo biloba* is remarkably resistant to all kinds of pollution, viruses, and fungi. For both biochemical reasons and because of its legendary resistance following the atomic bombings of Hiroshima and Nagasaki, it is one of the plants on which Mirko chose to focus his attention. Although Asian cultures have used ginkgo seeds medicinally for hundreds of years, the modern Western use of ginkgo is limited exclusively to the leaf. The green leaves of the tree are usually harvested from trees growing in plantations in South Korea, Japan, and France.

Green leaf extracts of *Ginkgo biloba* are commercially available everywhere as "standard preparations." The standardized green leaf extract is expected to contain about 24 percent flavoglycosides and 10 percent quercetin, which are recommended to improve circulation in the arteries, capillaries, veins, or within the brain.

Mirko's unique extract of *Ginkgo biloba* has very different properties from all other extracts on the market today, due to the time at which it is harvested and the particular extraction procedure.[12]

Only a few years earlier in 1967, Drs. M. V. Sirsat and S. S. Shrikhande reported that approximately 25 percent of radiation burns cause tumors, and that the lowered immunity resulting from radiation and/or chemotherapy predispose to malignant degeneration.[13]

Dr. John W. Gofman, professor emeritus of molecular and cellular biology at the University of California, Berkeley, conducted a large-scale investigation involving scientists, doctors, etiologists, and physicians. Gofman has been steadfast in advancing the notion that routine procedures such as fluoroscopy at hospitals throughout the nation, among a generation of children, exposed tens of thousands of patients to incredibly dangerous radiation levels that later resulted in cancers. Later, Gofman would charge that routine screening of premenopausal women with unintentionally high radiation levels would result in breast cancer excesses, and many epidemiological studies have shown increases among premenopausal women and cancer linked with screening (as opposed to diagnostic use of radiation). Essentially, everyone in the industrialized world is being exposed to radiation. Published in November 1999, the investigation entitled, "Radiation from Medical Procedures in the Pathogenesis of Cancer and Ischemic Heart Disease" found that "Medical radiation, introduced as a treatment in 1996, is becoming a factor in approximately half of all fatal cases of cancer in the U.S. The proof cited in my 1999 monograph, which no one has refuted, indicated that approximately 250,000 people in the U.S. die prematurely each year from cancer and coronary diseases, with half the cases due to the unnecessary and excessive use of X-rays that they received over a lifetime."

Radiation induces burns and alters ribonucleases (the enzymes which process RNA molecules). In a healthy cell, the normal function of these enzymes is to edit the genetic messages copied from the DNA, a process that is essential for overall good health. Often, these enzymes become deregulated or disrupted. Ultimately, this can have a damaging effect on the health of cells and connective tissues. It is therefore essential to protect the skin from burns, whether from the sun or from ionizing radiation, and regulate those enzymes.

Radiation-induced fibrosis is the late-developing effect of ionizing radiation. The scar tissue that forms as a result of radiation is insidious, and may not develop until 6 to 12 months or more after radiation. Although the mortality rate is low, suffering and subsequent complications are frequent. It is therefore important to protect the body during and for several months following ionizing radiation treatments, due to the slow appearance of fibrosis. The late onset of pulmonary and cardiac effects is also a common side effect of ionizing radiation, which in turn, is amplified by chemotherapy.

Mirko demonstrated in several experiments that his original ginkgo extract, through its regulatory or normalizing effect on cellular enzymes, helps the tissues to remain in good health, even when they are exposed to extreme physiological stresses.

Mirko showed that in many, if not all, fibrosis cases there are changes in nucleases that are linked to collagen production. This may explain how his unique *Ginkgo biloba* extract protected the skin from burns, inhibited scar formation, protected against fibrosis and also regulated the activity of several enzymes.

Mirko also demonstrated that skin cells exposed to radiation exhibit excessive RNase activity: Extracts from the exposed tissue quickly degraded normal (full length) RNA molecules into smaller fragments that lose their biological function. However, when Mirko added his purified *Ginkgo biloba* fraction, the excessive RNase activity was reversed and the full length RNA molecules persisted at their normal length (see Figures 4 and 5, page 58). This *Ginkgo biloba* preparation is an impressive example of a natural biological regulator that suppresses the abnormal activity of enzymes induced by radiation or other agents.

In another important study, mice received, either before or after being irradiated, different amounts of RNA fragments or golden leaf ginkgo extract. Autopsies were performed, organs were checked as well as survival rates, weight, and double-strand chromosome breaks (karyotypes). As shown in Figure 6 (page 58), those animals receiving both the RNA fragments and the Ginkgo lived much longer.

They survived their treatments better. Some results were published, but many other results were never published, due to the Army's procedures regarding classified information.

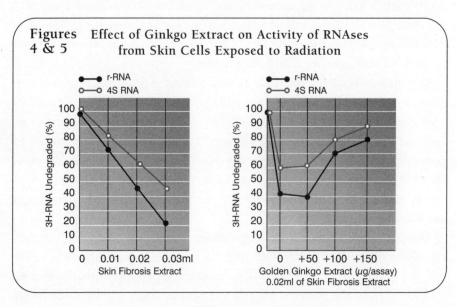

Figures 4 & 5 — Effect of Ginkgo Extract on Activity of RNAses from Skin Cells Exposed to Radiation

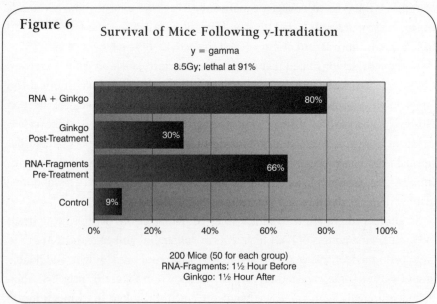

Figure 6 — Survival of Mice Following γ-Irradiation

The interest generated by the results of radioprotection led Mirko and a colleague to meet with a representative of the French atomic submarine base in Brest. They were hoping to awaken his interest for the benefit of the sailors, as it was well known that sailors living in atomic submarines are subjected to radiation and sometimes develop certain types of cancers (that can also be carried over to their sons or daughters via germ-line genetic damage). But the response was unexpected to the surprisingly naïve team. There was simply no way that the French military would admit any responsibility for cancers generated by radiation exposure. Consequently, they were not interested in any treatment whatsoever.

The Beljanski team remained at the Châtenay Malabry School of Pharmacy for 10 years. Then in 1988, Mirko reached retirement age and he had to stop working in accordance with French law. Mirko could not give up his work; research was his passion and his driving force in life. What was to become of the Beljanskis?

CHAPTER SIX

The Discovery of Destabilized DNA

Some months later, a French businessman, Pierre Silvestri, and his consorts came to speak with Mirko at his apartment in Paris. The businessman had just lost his son to leukemia and decided, along with a newly formed group for people suffering from various illnesses, to organize a research center in the south of France.

The group's financial supporter had purchased an unkempt but nonetheless beautiful property in Isère, south of Lyons, near the Burgundy region of France in a small village called St. Prim. Their desire was to focus on Beljanski's therapeutic concepts, anticancer and antiviral remedies.

Enlisting assistance from both Beljanskis, the businessman set about restoring the property with a youth association largely made up of recovering drug addicts. Many of the group's young people, who had been heavy drug users, were affected by Acquired Immune Deficiency Syndrome (AIDS).

By the following year, and for the first time in his life, Mirko had a beautiful, well-equipped private laboratory without the hindrances of a bureaucratic government institution, such as the Pasteur Institute. So, with two biochemistry graduate students and two well-trained technicians, he set about performing experiments on treatments for cancer, viral diseases, and immune diseases.

Pierre Silvestri said he would take charge of all the management. Mirko would only have to dedicate himself to research. Monique decided to stay in Paris where the couple had bought a modest location where she would be preparing the RNA fragments.

The surroundings were superb. Mirko, who was a nature lover, used to enjoy taking evening walks in the nearby tree-lined park. He had a sleeping room onsite and ate his meals in a small inn adjacent to the laboratory. Throughout the eight years he spent at his new laboratory, Mirko enjoyed the peace and quiet of the place. It was a period of fruitful research and calm. From it came a vast amount of theoretical and investigative as well as practical findings that would prove of great importance to people's health and the ability of the body to engage in reparative processes. Salaries and lab expenses were covered by the sale of products known as "préparations magistrales," which are customized preparations made for an individual patient by a pharmacist.

He now had peace, assistants, and nature. He was already very much involved in helping humanity. The team wanted to develop a cure for what was then a completely new disease: AIDS; and also broaden the approach with respect to cancer treatments and degenerative autoimmune diseases. From the eight years spent at his new laboratory in Isère came a vast amount of investigative findings and truly viable findings to support his approach to degenerative and infectious viral diseases.

And he never tired of learning and working.

The group's desire was to help Mirko take his molecular concepts, particularly his work with RNA, to the patient and to help in cases of cancer or the newly emerging acquired immune deficiency syndrome that was terrifying the world. If Mirko would develop tools that could be used and marketed, then there would be profits for everybody.

Even without the prestige of the Pasteur Institute, Mirko continued to turn out publications in the major scientific peer-reviewed journals and press. Always very active, the small team continued to develop other aspects of their research. New ideas about the initiation of cancer and its mechanisms had germinated in Mirko's mind during the long studies on plant cancer induction or arrest with various molecules. But one has to remember that the only explanation for the appearance of cancer was mutations, despite the fact that at that time analytic techniques did not show any constant appearance of a significant difference between healthy cell DNA and cancer cell DNA. But if there is more to cancer than just mutations, then what was it?

What Mirko conceived now was how the environment spoke to DNA. There were two ways: through reverse transcriptase, which he had discovered, or by directly attacking the very structure of the DNA and changing its spacial conformation.

As he had first noticed during his long research on plants and the cancerization process, DNA needs a change of its three-dimensional structure right before the oncogenic RNA initiates the cancer cells. He had seen that this destabilization process of the DNA is accomplished by the plant hormones before cancer induction by RNA. This destabilization of the DNA's double helix created the right conditions for modification of DNA's function. This mechanism led him to study the class of compounds acting as promoters or procarcinogens. In fact, they provoke biochemical and cumulative changes to the double-helix structure. The damage to the DNA conformation is the beginning of the downfall of the cell.

His first goal was to examine the difference between DNAs that were isolated and purified from normal versus cells known to be cancerous. He observed different rates of DNA duplication which correspond to changes in the physical helical structure of the DNA rather than at the level of the genetic content of the DNA. (The identity of the nucleotides at successive positions along the DNA polymer is known as a DNA sequence.) Obtaining this information is the central goal of the human genome project in order to find the critical differences between the DNA sequences of normal and malignant cells.

In complete contrast to this approach, Mirko sought to identify the differences between normal and cancer DNAs at the level of the physical structure of the double-stranded DNA by testing for changes in the stability of the double helix. He used various assays to show that the special conformation of DNA from cancer cells is different from the DNA of normal cells. He measured the difference in absorption of ultraviolet (UV) light by the two DNA types, which indicates how tightly the two strands of DNA are held together in the double helix; the greater the strand separation, the higher the absorption of UV. He conceived of DNA not as a mathematician but as an artist and physicist. This was remarkable.

The absorption of DNA from cancer cells was consistently higher (by 1 to 5 percent) than the results found for normal DNAs and correlated with the more rapid speed of DNA duplication in cancer cells as well as the cell multiplication rate. He always studied all these aspects in comparison with healthy DNAs or tissues. But in the presence of carcinogens (Mirko used all known potent carcinogens) the two strands of DNA from cancer cells were always immediately separated (up to 30 percent), while the strands of the healthy cell DNA remained almost unchanged. Destabilization of DNA in a healthy cell requires the persistent and cumulative effect of carcinogens, a result which cannot be seen in a quick *in vitro* test. Thirty to 40 percent is almost the maximum opening for DNA; a point of destabilization where the DNA is no longer metabolically active. Mirko concluded that the chemical bonds that hold the double helix together are reproductibly disrupted in cancer DNA, which results in more openings or loops than are present in normal DNA; this was confirmed by the melting point. He referred to this pattern of relaxation in certain portions of DNA of cancer cells as "destabilization."

The opening and closing of the DNA helix in cells is part of the dynamic of life: Whenever the DNA replicates or when the information it contains is expressed, the strands must be separated to enable access of the enzymatic machinery that perform duplication and transcription. In a healthy cell, the opening of the DNA is well-regulated and the loops are re-closed when these processes are complete. The persistent openings Beljanski found in cancer DNA could be the cause of the deregulation of DNA metabolism that is the hallmark of most cancers: destabilization of the DNA structure allows for excess replication and aberrant gene expression. This suggested that if the DNA were, in fact, destabilized into frequent loops then it should serve as a more active template for its own duplication performed in the test tube than the more tightly wound duplexes characteristic of purified normal DNA. This prediction was confirmed in experiments demonstrating that cancer DNA replicated more rapidly than normal DNA as measured by the incorporation of specially labeled nucleotides into polymeric form. Given the exact same amount of DNA template, nucleotide building blocks, and the enzyme known as DNA polymerase, the reaction containing cancer DNA consistently synthesized more new DNA. Thus, DNA destabilization was correlated with enhanced DNA synthesis. All these phenomena were extensively verified with healthy and cancerous DNAs issued from many different sources, including plants, mammals, and humans.

What had Beljanski accomplished? Like any research scientist who focuses on cancer, he looked for a fundamental difference between cancer cells and normal cells. He identified this difference as an alteration in the helical structure of cancer DNA—not at the level of mutations in the DNA sequence—but in disruptions of the DNA double strands. He devised a simple laboratory test, which he called the Oncotest, for identifying compounds that could cause and promote *in vitro* the destabilization of DNA. He showed that all known carcinogens acted in exactly this way (as shown in Figures 7-10, pages 65-66).

Figure 7

What Happens in the Presence of a Carcinogen

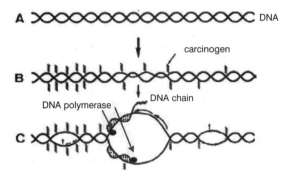

Once the strands are separated, enzymes for DNA replication have increased access to the duplication sites located inside the double helix and duplication can become abnormally accelerated.

Figure 8

Beljanski's Theory of Cancer

• The primary structure of DNA relates to how the nucleotides of each strand line up with each other.

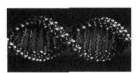

Mutations = modifications in one or more nucleotides.

• Secondary structure of DNA relates to how the two DNA strands line up via hydrogen bonding.

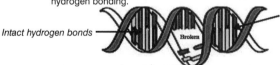

Intact hydrogen bonds

Intact hydrogen bonds —

Broken

Beljanski's Theory is that **cancer DNA differs from normal DNA in its secondary structure**, rather than only its primary structure.

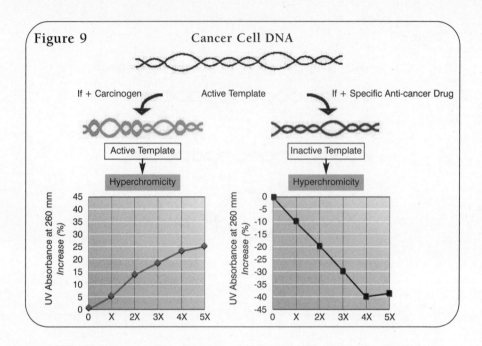

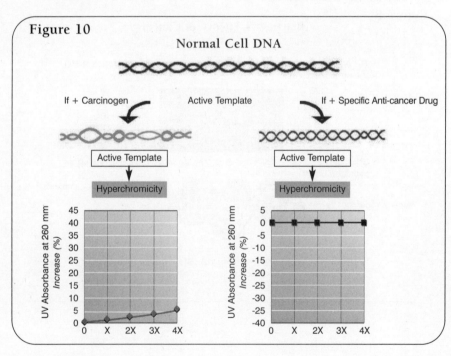

The Oncotest (see Figure 11) is a fast *in vitro* test that shows the strong amplification of cancer-DNA synthesis in the presence of carcinogenic molecules while the rate of DNA synthesis from healthy cells is only slightly increased. The stimulation of cancer DNA synthesis is due to the destabilization that all carcinogens immediately induce in the conformation of cancer DNA.

In the course of his experiments with the Oncotest, Mirko discovered to his surprise that numerous agents, not normally considered as carcinogenic substances,

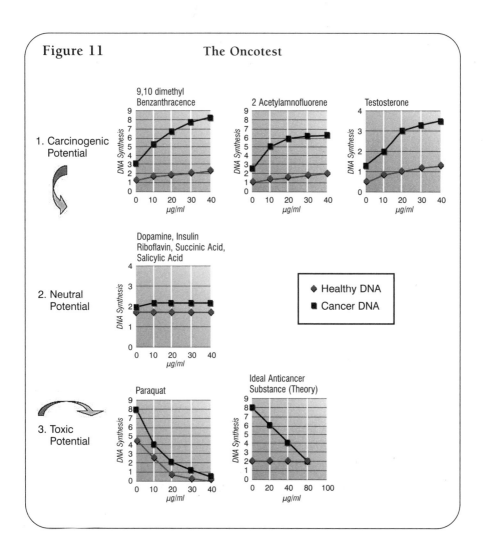

Figure 11   **The Oncotest**

behaved like well-known carcinogens. For example, as illustrated in Figure 12, certain antibiotics, anti-inflammatories, low doses of chemotherapy, radiation or hormones could combine to cause greater cumulative damage to the secondary structure.

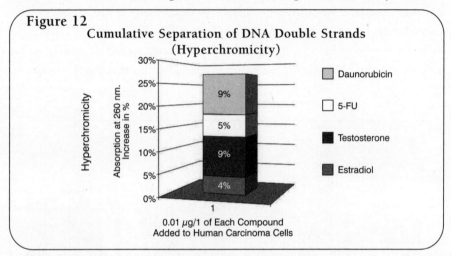

Figure 12

Cumulative Separation of DNA Double Strands (Hyperchromicity)

Once Mirko became convinced of how reliable the Oncotest was, he decided to approach pharmaceutical groups, hoping to get them interested and have them use it to warrant the quality of their products. The Oncotest was sensitive, fast, low-priced and extremely reliable. Again, their response was predictable. Too much knowledge about the toxicity of their own chemicals was not a good thing according to their companies' business models.

Nobody was interested. It could have been a remarkable prevention tool to slow down the enormous progression of cancer cases all over the world due to pollution. To the contrary, for the pharmaceutical and industrial chemical complex it would be far better that the test be suppressed. It was bad for business.

A new scientific opportunity presented itself. It was basic logic: If all substances with a carcinogenic potential stimulate the synthesis of cancer DNA and not healthy DNA, maybe substances exist that do exactly the opposite and that are capable of inhibiting the cancer DNA duplication but not that of healthy DNA.

He then went on to use this test to search for compounds with effects that were the opposite of carcinogens. In his work with these compounds, Mirko created new perspectives for cancer phytotherapy and selective anticancer agents that would act much like a scalpel in the body by acting only against cancer DNA or specifically against cancer DNA, rather than like the ax of chemotherapy and radiation. He had begun to implement the concept of selectively targeted cancer treatments that left healthy cells alone.

He found some alkaloids such as alstonine or sempervirine (or flavopereirine), when isolated and purified, strongly inhibited the *in vitro* synthesis of cancerous DNA, practically without affecting the synthesis of normal DNA. Moreover, they were capable of thwarting the destabilizing effect of carcinogens. Therefore, they should be able to prevent *in vivo* both the development of malignant tumors and the transformation of a normal cell into a cancerous cell.

In particular, the team focused on screening natural compounds, not just because of their diversity, but because he reasoned that natural compounds would be more physiologic to use as anticancer agents in humans.

Beljanski frequently expressed a total rejection of toxic substances. "Never would I be able to sleep," he told his wife, "if I gave animals or people, who put their trust in me, substances that have the potential to be toxic."

The team focused on two plants of the Apocynaceae family, *Rauwolfia vomitoria* and Pao pereira.

Mirko and his researchers demonstrated that both plant extracts enter environmentally damaged and susceptible cells much more effectively than they enter normal cells. In other words, they are selective (see Figures 13 and 14 on the following page).

When the cell becomes cancerous, the porosity of its membrane changes, which allows all kinds of molecules, good or bad, to penetrate cancer cells. When the plant extract penetrates the cancer cell, the DNA can no longer duplicate or renew itself, and the cell dies.

The team had to show that, once the plant extract penetrated the cancer cell, it acted the same way as it did on purified DNA. In other words, the team had to isolate and characterize the active principle of the two plants, control their activity, both *in vitro* and *in vivo*, find good purification processes, and make sure they were not toxic for healthy cells. It was a lot of work, and it kept them very busy for a long time.

Many chemotherapy drugs like vinblastine, vincristine, or taxol derivatives are based on a synthetic copy of natural molecules, but they are very toxic to healthy cells because their mode of action is not selective.

The effects of the Rauwolfia and Pao pereira extracts had first been studied in plants. In fact, earlier, working with Dr. L. Le Goff and M. I. Aaron-da-Cunha gave

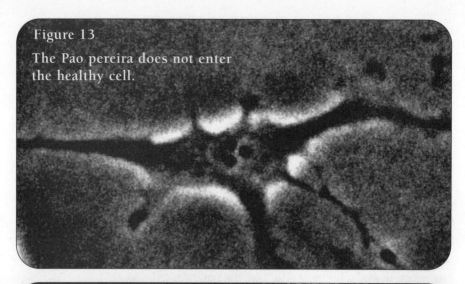

Figure 13

The Pao pereira does not enter the healthy cell.

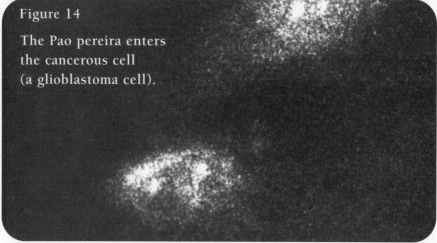

Figure 14

The Pao pereira enters the cancerous cell (a glioblastoma cell).

the Beljanskis the opportunity to verify the effect of Pao pereira and Rauwolfia extracts on plants also suffering from cancer or viral attacks. Later, it was fascinating to discover that all the results obtained in plants could be applied to a great variety of cells *in vitro*, then to other living biological systems, and, much later, to humans.

These experiments, including toxicology tests by experts, took place over a period of 10 years, but the Rauwolfia and Pao pereira extracts proved to be almost universal opponents to cells with destabilized DNA.

Mirko quickly thought of a way to improve the *in vivo* results by combining a very light conventional treatment with the Rauwolfia or the Pao treatment. Why? Because in low dosages, antimitotics and radiotherapy destabilize cancerous DNA and spread its strands apart as previously shown, thus laying bare additional initiation sites where the alkaloids can bind. This would enhance the binding of anticancer molecules and thus would improve the efficacy of their action. In fact, there is a real additive effect, a synergy between the classical drugs used in cancer treatment and the plant alkaloids. The team administered very low doses of both the Rauwolfia extract and of antimitotics (i.e., the chemotherapy drug CCNU [Lomustine], one of the older chemotherapeutic agents, which has been in use for many years and is taken orally as a capsule). While all the control animals were dead by the 30th day, the survival rate for those treated only with Rauwolfia was 30 percent at 90 days, and for those treated only with the chemotherapy drug survival was 45 percent at 90 days. But when the two treatments (plant extract + Lomustine) were combined, the survival rate reached 100 percent (see Figures 15 and 16).

Many other similar tests were conducted combining Rauwolfia or Pao pereira extract with various chemotherapeutic agents such as 5FU, Endoxan, and daunorubicin. Numerous experiments showed that plant extracts do not attach to normal DNA and had no toxicity *in vivo*, especially with regard to the fragile blood cells. The animals that recovered survived in excellent health and suffered neither weight loss nor other undesirable side effects. Both plant extracts also minimized the usual harmful effects of antimitotics and radiotherapy.

The table on page 73 (Figure 17) shows a list of lines of cells that have been destroyed by the presence of Pao pereira extract, as demonstrated by Mirko's research. This was published posthumously, in 2000 in the journal *Genetic and Molecular Biology* (23:29-33).

However, to make the table clearer, we have recalculated the results as percent of inhibition after 48 hours of incubation in the presence of 100 µg/ml of extract. Different laboratories have conducted several toxicology experiments confirming the remarkable innocuity of these plant extracts in the presence of healthy cells.

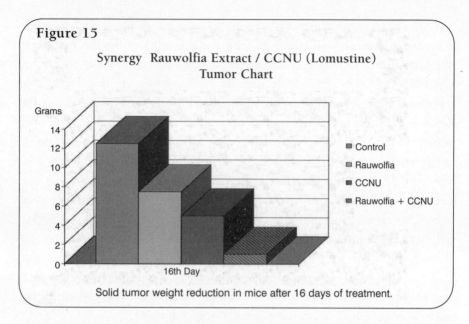

Figure 15

Synergy Rauwolfia Extract / CCNU (Lomustine)
Tumor Chart

Solid tumor weight reduction in mice after 16 days of treatment.

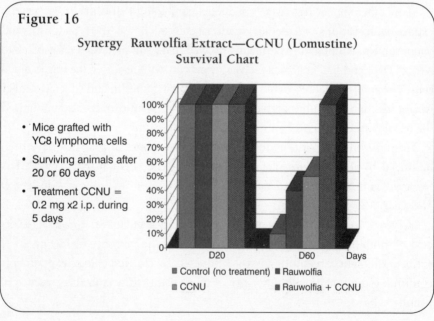

Figure 16

Synergy Rauwolfia Extract—CCNU (Lomustine)
Survival Chart

- Mice grafted with YC8 lymphoma cells
- Surviving animals after 20 or 60 days
- Treatment CCNU = 0.2 mg x2 i.p. during 5 days

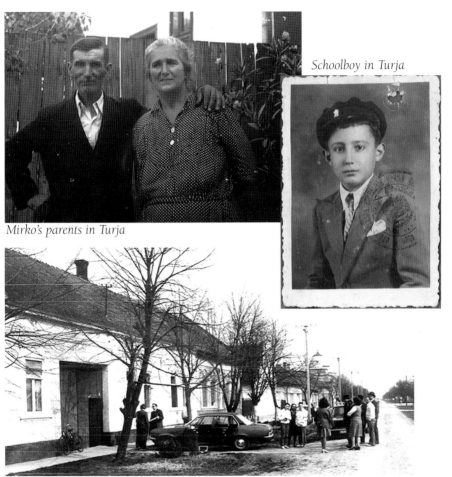

Schoolboy in Turja

Mirko's parents in Turja

Turja, where Mirko studied as a teen

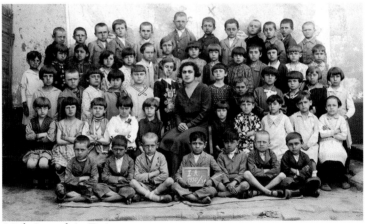

Mirko's youth in Turja

Mirko and Monique wedding 1951

Newlyweds

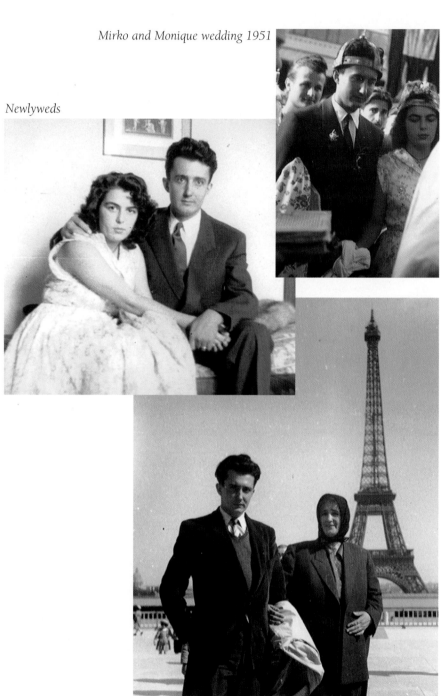

Mirko in Paris with his mother, June 1952, at the Eiffel Tower

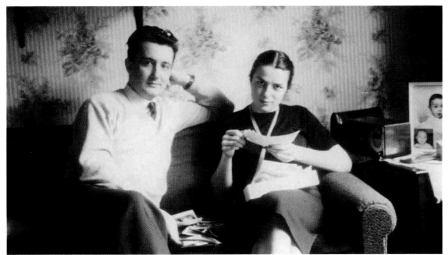

Monique and Mirko 1956

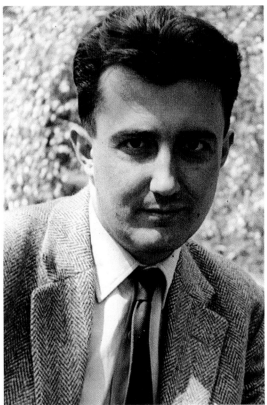

Spring 1956

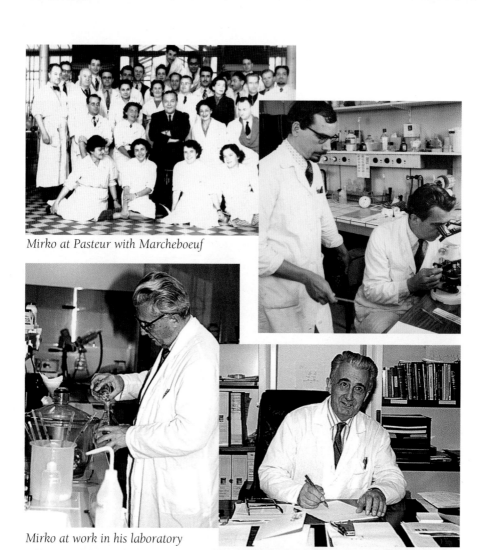

Mirko at Pasteur with Marcheboeuf

Mirko at work in his laboratory

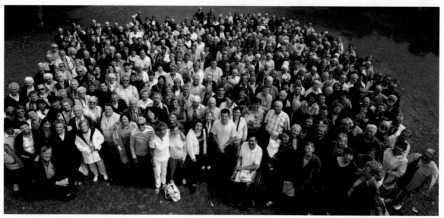

Cancer survivors gather for an annual day-long picnic in Saintes, France. They credit their success to Mirko Beljanski's formulations.

During the clinical observations, it was also noted by doctors that both alkaloid extracts seemed to have helped their patients cope better with the extreme toxicity and physiological stress of their allopathic regimens.

All these results were excellent and demonstrated the advantage of combining the two types of treatment. But the real test came with people who were not finding satisfactory help with the conventional treatments offered through the European medical system.

Figure 17

Cancer Cell Inhibition by the Beljanski Molecules

Cancer	Cell Type	% Inhibition
Brain	U 251	99.64
	CCF-STTG-1	97.71
	SW 1088	97.82
	C6	94.04
Colon	LoVo	95.35
	CaCo-2	95.26
Liver	Sk-Hep 1	94.48
Kidney	A 498	95.66
Skin	G-361	96.61
Ovary	ES 2	97.86
	SW 626	95.57
Breast	ZR-75-1	83.78
	MCF-7	89.76
Pancreas	MIA PaCa2	97.41
Prostate thyroid	PC3	85.28
	TT	91.17

Under the same *in vitro* conditions, **normal cell lines**
(brain, colon, liver, kidney and ovary) were not destroyed.

In early 1982, only a couple years from retirement, Jean Le Guen began to experience digestive problems—the first signs of what would turn out to be a "long and cruel" disease.

"Wanting to quickly discover the cause of these problems, I saw a general practitioner. From there, I went from specialist to specialist until the diagnosis was finally confirmed by a biopsy. The conclusion unfortunately was pessimistic: It confirmed the existence of a malignant pancreatic tumor."

In March, Le Guen, a small farmer well-known in Finistère for his activities pertaining to unions, was, after a biopsy, diagnosed with a cancerous tumor of the pancreas (adenocarcinoma) that was resistant to chemotherapy and radiation. Jean was not young, and the hospital gave very little hope to his wife Marguerite.

Says Le Guen, "The tumor could not be removed and appeared to be both chemotherapy and radiation resistant. My wife asked the doctor, 'What can we do?' His response was simple: 'Well, nothing, Ma'am.' She then asked how long I had left, to which he responded, 'Two months, three months, maybe more, maybe less.'"

His wife had heard of Mirko's work and the new treatment being spoken about. On her extreme insistence, the head of the hospital in Brest asked Mirko for the Pao and Rauwolfia extracts.

The team had already been assured of the nontoxicity of the products, but they had not yet crossed the threshold of giving the products to humans.

However, faced with Jean's desperate situation and the official request from the hospital, Mirko and Monique decided to send Jean some capsules of the Pao pereira and *Rauwolfia vomitoria* extracts, as well as an extract of *Ginkgo biloba* to protect him from the rays that were administered to him in weak doses. The tumor became radiation-sensitive and, in the presence of the alkaloids, decreased in size.

As Le Guen explained, "The concrete results of the treatment were apparent on two levels: first, the tumor was halted in its initial form, and, second, the initial resistance of the tumor was modified, causing it to finally respond to traditional hospital treatments. Over the course of the next year, there were highs and lows, but all of it was with a minimum of suffering."

Le Guen regained his health completely. He lived to be an old man, and in 2006, offered this testimony that he confirmed again in 2008, "Even after completing radiation therapy, I continued with the Beljanski products (Pao, Rauwolfia,

Ginkgo biloba and RNA Fragments) for several years in maintenance doses until 1985 when I went off them completely. It has been 24 years and I have been in good health ever since."

Because Le Guen was very well-known in Bretagne, this success had a lively response, and soon numerous demands from doctors and patients bombarded the team. "We were not equipped to handle this demand, but at the same time, we were consumed with curiosity to know just how much we could help these people and what the limits of the products were," recalled Monique.

Soon Mirko's team was flooded with requests from desperate patients and they started giving away the precious capsules to the extent that they could. They enjoyed helping people and also were very interested in observing what the extracts could actually do and the extent of their efficacy.

One day, in 1986, Mirko received a phone call from Gérard Weidlich, a gendarme, who was only 40. Weidlich told Mirko, "I live on the Atlantic coast. I have been contaminated by the HIV virus. Nothing can help me."

(At this time, AZT was not yet available.) "My doctor heard through a friend that you have a substance active against viruses."

"But we only tested its antiviral properties on plants and mice!" Mirko replied.

"I'll hop on the train and come to see you," said the man.

"I want to save my life, I want to try it. I have a wife and four kids to raise. I already have opportunistic infections, and no matter what, there is nothing else," the patient stated.

Mirko hesitated, torn between the desire to help him and the fear to disappoint him if the product failed. The patient insisted, got the capsules and gave Mirko a discharge letter. In fact the Pao pereira extract had been tested for various antiviral activities and was a good candidate to fight viral disease. The fact that it has no toxic side effects was also a reason to respond to his request.

Fifteen days later, Weidlich already felt much better. He lived 20 more years in great shape. He became president of the CIRIS association that defends the rights of patients who wish to augment their treatment with complementary medicine and natural health products.

In the course of his research, Mirko had previously demonstrated that the Pao pereira extract had an inhibitive effect on reverse transcriptase, the enzyme by which the HIV virus can multiply within the cell. As plants are often infected by RNA viruses, they are a convenient model to demonstrate that Pao inhibits this type of

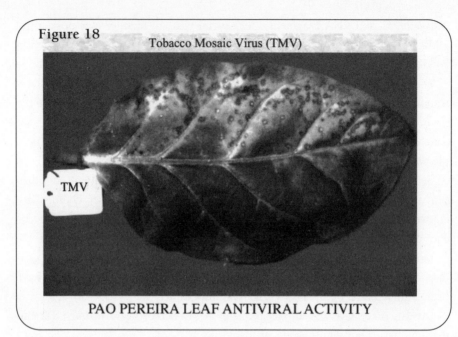

Figure 18

Tobacco Mosaic Virus (TMV)

TMV

PAO PEREIRA LEAF ANTIVIRAL ACTIVITY

virus. The results were excellent (see an example of RNA-related damage in plants in Figure 18).

The interest in the Beljanski products was growing in the French population. Many patients became aware of the research concerning these specific plant molecules and RNA fragments. The Beljanskis received many requests from patients and doctors but did not have the means to meet the demand for his substances.

France possesses a highly technological Big Pharma-oriented medical health care system. For the most part, drugs which have toxic side-effects are accepted by the official health authorities, but little else is eligible for government-funded health care or widely available, and health care professionals have much less freedom of therapeutic choice than in the United States. Even though there was and still remains a strong opposition to complementary and alternative medicine (CAM) and natural medicine, there has always been an undercurrent of naturopathy or natural medicine. While enzyme preparations, mistletoe and other natural medicines are highly touted in Germany as a means of supplementing cancer treatment programs, these never made their way into France. If some natural medicines were sold or prescribed in France, it was always with difficulties and aggressiveness from the medical authorities against the medical doctor, no matter how well-qualified, and even against patients who preferred them as part of their human rights within the scope of medical and health freedom. Despite all those difficulties, a growing legion of doctors learned about Mirko's work through his proliferating publications, patients, and conferences.

During all these years, Mirko maintained close working relationships with doctors and scientists in Europe who liked him.

Mirko was fully aware of the potential difficulties his products might encounter with health officials, but the results and the satisfaction of patients incited him to go forward. Patients did not suffer to the same degree the usual ravages, such as nausea, loss of hair or harm to the blood cells, when they used combined approach of allopathic medicine with the supportive RNA fragments and plant molecules. The concomitant use of the Beljanski approach, alone or with the procedures and medicines of the medical bureaucracy, seemed to many patients to help. Quality of life was in almost all cases greatly improved.

Despite these obstacles, more and more doctors began prescribing the Beljanski products for their patients, some of whom wanted to use such therapies exclusively. They yielded beneficial effects in most cases. Numerous more patients wanted to combine the plant molecules for health reasons with conventional treatments, while still others took them regularly as preventive measures to maintain health.

CASE STUDIES

GEORGES CHAOUI had much of his prostate removed in 1986 at age 64. Unfortunately in 1991 during a medical follow-up by the Department of Urology, Bordeaux University Hospital Center, tumors were discovered in his bladder and the remaining part of his prostate. Given this diagnosis, his doctors in both Bordeaux and Paris suggested chemotherapy with a BCG drip. He thus underwent BCG drips at various frequencies for one year. However, his doctors didn't know that in addition to these drips he was taking six capsules daily of Rauwolfia extract.

Twelve years later, he testified, "Thus, I am here today to attest to the efficacy of the Beljanski products, and in particular, the Rauwolfia extract. Medical statements made by my doctor at the Bordeaux University Hospital Center in 1995 reinforce my own comments. And the doctor (not knowing I had taken the Beljanski products) concluded with a nod of his head, 'Yes, it's a miracle!'"

To avoid any possible relapse, he said he continued to take three capsules daily of Rauwolfia extract and three capsules of Pao pereira. "As part of my medical follow-up, the doctors have observed that I even have a regrowth of normal prostate tissue."

M. RONAN LANNUZEL was diagnosed with lymphoblastic lymphoma (a serious form of leukemia) in 1987 and was hospitalized at the University Hospital Center receiving chemotherapy as his main treatment. Following that, he chose to have a bone marrow transplant rather than continuing chemotherapy whose duration no one could predict. Throughout the entire period, he used the Beljanski products as a supplement to his treatment.

"My physicians were surprised to see how fast my white blood cells returned— on the ninth day after the transplant rather than on the 21st day as is commonly the case. And my departure from the hospital came more than a month before their earliest prediction.

"There was an enormous difference in my response to treatment versus those of other patients treated in the same way—but without the aid of the Beljanski products. I continue to take these supplements two to three times per year as a maintenance treatment. For 12 years now, to the great astonishment of my friends who thought my situation was hopeless, I have led a completely normal life."

STRICKEN WITH MYELOMA, discovered in September of 1988, Ernest Morteau's wife underwent very heavy chemotherapy treatments for four years. The side effects of these treatments led to two aplasias at the beginning of 1989 and resulted in her being transferred to intensive care in a coma. Her immune defenses were extremely weak and the doctor's prognosis was quite bleak. Said her husband Ernest, "I don't think she could have survived these tests had she not received the help" of the Beljanski molecules in time, ensuring the repair of various cellular anomalies and quickly re-establishing her immune system defenses. For more than 15 years, she has been monitored with traditional medicine. "Seasonal check-ups show a level of stabilization that surprises those in the medical field, especially for a person stricken with this type of cancer. Since 1993, she has had no further need for treatment. However, she continues to benefit from the Beljanski products, which I am sure have provided this stability. The proof of their effectiveness? In 2007, she is alive and still doing well."

YVON PAPINEAU had no idea what it meant to be sick until age 65. He noticed, to his distress, that one of his testicles was progressively getting larger to the point of doubling in volume, while becoming hard to the touch. He started to worry and consulted a doctor. Papineau was sent to a specialist in Royan, who, after examining him, kept him there for three days during which time it became necessary to have the testicle removed. The operation was necessary, according to him, because without it, "The problem would have proved fatal within two months."

Yet he still had a lymphoma. After 18 months of chemotherapy "drips" and radiation "waves," "the doctors told him, 'You're cured!'"

Everything was going well until the summer of 1995 when he suffered a lung infection. A short time afterward, he had an enormous growth in his throat. After a series of incorrect diagnoses, the specialist made the decision to operate at Rochefort. The excised tumor was analyzed and it turned out to be non-Hodgkin's lymphoma. He was immediately sent to Bordeaux for three days of tests.

On the advice of friends, he went for his first time to a doctor familiar with the Beljanski products. "I very quickly noticed the competence of the homeopathic doctor who surprised me when he told me I had to follow the protocol prescribed by the oncologists because it was vital as well. However, he suggested prescribing the new Beljanski products for me, which would allow me to better endure the very heavy treatments. For one thing, he said the chemotherapy treatments would no longer need to be interrupted because of the loss of white blood cells."

He started the Beljanski treatment and, in his own testimony stated he "was much better able to withstand the chemotherapy and radiation therapy sessions." He added that, "in comparison with a sick friend, afflicted with the same illness and who didn't use Beljanski products, I figure that I came out pretty well. He lost 20 kilograms and [was] completely devastated physically."

Another surgery was necessary to remove the catheter. At that point, he was also taking Pao pereira and the golden leaf ginkgo extract. "When I came back to see the specialists four days before the date assigned for removing the stitches, seeing the speed and perfect healing that had taken place, I heard the reaction which by then had become familiar: 'That's incredible!'"

He commented, "In my head, I tell myself that I'm in a cycling race and that, up until now, it's been all uphill. With the help of Beljanski products, I'm still hanging in there and I've gotten over the worst of it. The most difficult part is over, and it can only get easier on the descent.

"Nowadays, I feel better and better. I came out of this thanks to the Beljanski products. My illness taught me one simple thing that most people haven't yet realized: How beautiful life is!"

IN THE 1990S, JEAN-PAUL LEPERLIER discovered Dr. Beljanski's products. "The first time I came across Dr. Beljanski's products was not as a sick person, but as a journalist carrying out an investigation against Mirko Beljanski.

"He had been described to me as a quack pretending to cure all sorts of diseases with fake medicines. My goal was to find 20 or so 'victims' who had taken Beljanski's products who would testify against the pseudo-scientist for providing them with harmful medication. Despite months of effort, I was not able to find anyone with complaints. And then, unable to believe it, I was stricken with cancer of the intestine. I allowed the tumor to grow excessively, which led to an extreme diagnosis: 'You have three months to live, and they will be three months of hell,' my doctor told me.

"Ironically, I decided to try the products I had set out to discredit. Protected by Beljanski's unique ginkgo extract, I was able to endure radiation therapy at extremely high dosages. As my DNA was destabilized by the aggressiveness of the radiation, I used Pao pereira and *Rauwolfia vomitoria*. The key phrase in Beljanski's approach that comes to mind is 'synergy of action.' Lastly, my immune defenses, decimated by chemotherapy, were able to recover because of the RNA fragments. Years have passed, and I'm alive and still doing well in the fall of 2008."

For nearly a decade, Beljanski's molecules were dispensed not only in France but also Belgium, Switzerland, and Italy, among other nations. Many thousands of patients took his extracts. He had never advertised or publicized the molecules or his work except in peer-reviewed journals, but people were writing him and telling him that the products were helping them. The word of mouth worked wonders. The Beljanskis could not meet the public demand on their own. In France, herbal and other natural formulas and their manufacture must be approved before they are allowed to be sold in the marketplace. The Beljanski team applied for official French authorization called the Autorisation de Mise sur le Marché, the equivalent of FDA Approval in the United States.

But Mirko had more ominous enemies within the government. On the other hand, the officials at the Pasteur Institute were also angry at the popular success met by the Beljanski products.

The French authorities began to close in on Mirko. An article by A. Dorozynski in the July 16, 1994, issue of the *British Medical Journal* (*BMJ*) reported that a "French antiviral drug is ruled ineffective."

The *BMJ* noted that French health authorities declared Beljanski's antiviral extract ineffective, yet one "that has been prescribed to hundreds of patients with AIDS over the past six years. The extract, Pao pereira, was designed by a former researcher at the Pasteur Institute, Mirko Beljanski, and has become increasingly popular with doctors and patients, although its prescription and marketing have never been authorized. A number of patients are still receiving it, and it is far from certain that the so called 'Beljanski affair' is over.

"Beljanski, a doctor of biology, joined the Pasteur Institute in 1948, when he was 25, to work under Professor Pierre Lépine, who developed the French polio vaccine. Later, he moved to the Molecular Biology Department and advanced the then-unorthodox hypothesis that RNA could also be transcribed into DNA. This was confirmed a few years later."

In fact, as early as 1989, Claude Evin, then minister of social affairs and health, filed charges of illicit practice of medicine against Beljanski. A French politician and lawyer, he had been deputy mayor of Saint-Nazaire, a post he held until 1989. In his lengthy career, he held a variety of positions including Vice President of the National Assembly (1986-87), Minister for Health (1988-91), and Minister for Social Affairs (1988-91). The ministry ordered the association of doctors who favored the production to cease promoting it and prohibited pharmacies from selling it.

In March, court who had jurisdiction over the laboratory decided that Beljanski was NOT guilty of the illegal practice of medicine and, in order to come up with some kind of civil sentence, commanded him to pay 1 Franc (about 1 dime) to the French "Ordre des Médecins" (National Board of Doctors). A few days later, police searched Mirko's laboratories and placed him, Alain Boquet (a director), and Pierre Silvestri (former chairman of the board of the association of doctors favoring the product) under investigation for illegal production and sales of a pharmaceutical product.

Beljanski was in trouble. His findings were being called into question in an inquest that a fair-minded person would have to doubt was hardly equitable in design or intent. In December 1993, Professor Jean-François Girard, General Director of Health, asked the national agency for research on AIDS to carry out a series of tests to verify the alleged activity of PB-100. By July 1994, Girard stated that the inquiry had found no evidence justifying the therapeutic use of PB-100 as an antiviral agent. The witch hunt was on.

However, there was deep suspicion by Monique that continues to this day that the French authorities and scientists adulterated the formula or simply performed a test meant to fail, as the same materials turned over to Professor Girard were tested separately and independently in Switizerland by another specialist. Dr. D. Jachertz was former head of the Institute for Medicine at the University of Bern. In a report the author obtained, this test clearly demonstrated the anti-viral activity of the Pao extract.

A small-time regional disciplinary branch of the French medical association examined charges made against a doctor in Lyons for prescribing the Beljanski formulas to patients with cancer and AIDS. However, throughout France, Switzerland, and elsewhere in Europe, doctors continued to prescribe the formulas.

"This was hard to bear," recalled Monique. "Only the results and the appreciation of his patients were able to lighten the burden for Mirko."

And then came a very special patient whose use of the molecules provided the Beljanskis with a much-needed reprieve from their persecution. What happened next quieted everyone. Just when the hounds had their quarry cornered, they would be called off and whimper away. No one could touch Mirko—for as long as the president of France lived.

CHAPTER SEVEN

Mitterrand

O f the many patients who swallowed Beljanski's capsules, there was one who stood out from the rest. On September 17, 1992, *The New York Times* announced that President François Mitterrand had prostate cancer. The doctors said they had found cancerous lesions in tissue taken from his prostate in surgery but the illness was not life-threatening. The 75-year-old French leader left Cochin Hospital vowing to stay in power, throwing into doubt France's referendum to join the European Union, which Mitterrand favored. A statement issued by Elysée Palace said he was recovering normally. Yet many persons in government hoped his disease would accelerate. By then, Mitterrand had been in power some 11 years and had many opponents.

By 1993, Mitterrand was seriously ill with poorly treated prostate cancer. He already had many metastases. Rumors began circulating in the press, feeding speculation about his chances of survival and possible successors. A published press photo of him at the time revealed an emaciated and ravaged man who seemed absolutely cadaverous.

Not long after the release of that startling photo, the administrative head of the hospital that was treating him announced the president would not be able to complete his term and that elections were anticipated. The hospital's medical doctors gave Mitterrand three months to live. A mad scramble began amidst media frenzy, with candidates offering to fill ministerial positions and other government jobs.

In truth, Mitterrand had been battling prostate cancer for a long time.[14] There were rumors in 1981 that Mitterrand was suffering from cancer after he entered the Val-de-Grâce military hospital under an assumed name. President Mitterrand denied the rumors in May 1982, describing his malady as lumbago. In fact, he was diagnosed soon after his election in 1981, but the secret was kept from the nation for more than 10 years, according to an article in the January 10, 1996, edition of *Le Monde*.

If the cancer was diagnosed in late 1981 or early 1982, as *Le Monde* said, the report left in doubt how much President Mitterrand himself knew about the seriousness of his illness. Having observed the obsessive secrecy that surrounded the final days of President Georges Pompidou, Mr. Mitterrand had promised transparency about the state of his own health. But, of course, that, too, was doublespeak.

Le Monde added that when the disease was first diagnosed, the cancer was already too advanced to operate, and doctors decided instead to treat the president with hormones and other medical therapies, which they did for a decade, according to its account. Actually, Mitterrand promised as a candidate to release regular bulletins about his health, and his illness was first revealed after an operation in September 1992, though by then it had already been a 10-year battle.[15]

The president's office lied and said then that the cancer had been caught at an early stage and would not impede the president from carrying out his functions, though others suspected it had already spread to his bones.[16] A routine official bulletin issued less than three months earlier, in July 1992, had said his health was normal.

In March 1988, Mitterrand ran for reelection and was reelected for a second seven year term. But the president was in a lot of pain due to the metastasis and the progression of the disease. He underwent surgery, which was performed by a very powerful man, the brother of the head of the French National Assembly. This surgeon, Dr. Bernard Debré, head of urology at Cochin Hospital, reported to the press that the president was "feeling fine."

For many years, Mitterrand led a double life; he had two families and a daughter who lived in a secret area of the Elysée Palace. The press was complicit in revealing nothing. Toward the end of 1994, when Mitterrand acknowledged that he was often in great pain, he began receiving radiation therapy.

His mistress, Anne Pingeon, had a friend, Dr. Philippe de Kuyper, a fully accredited medical doctor who knew about Beljanski's work. Anne Pingeon shared her concerns regarding the president's health with Dr. de Kuyper and asked him to pay the president a medical visit. They got along very well. Mitterrand felt comfortable when the doctor prescribed the Beljanski formulas.

But all remained a secret. Mitterrand's official doctors were upset by the arrival of not only de Kuyper but his recommendation of the Beljanski molecules. Yet Mitterrand's health improved. Shortly thereafter, President Mitterrand regained his appetite. His strength and vigor returned, and he reasserted his political authority. In eight weeks, he had gained a noticeable amount of weight, smiled more with the show of good cheer, and began to look quite healthy, all to the utter shock of the politicos.

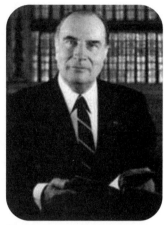

President Mitterrand appearing in good health after two months on the Beljanski molecules.

Knowing of the brewing rivalries and wishing not to stoke the fire, Dr. de Kuyper remained silent, as did the Beljanskis and Mitterrand. But the press toyed with Beljanski. On November 18, 1995, the weekly magazine *Le Point* No. 1209 published the following notice: "Distress in the office of Simone Weil (Health Minister): The medication taken by Mitterrand is going to be great publicity for natural products, and especially a not-yet-authorized product."

In reaction and to calm the brewing rivalries between the Elysée Palace's official doctors and this "insurgent," Mitterrand published a note in which he declared that the medication administered by Dr. de Kuyper had greatly helped him. The frenzy died down—for a time.

President Mitterrand was able to complete the 18 months of his second term. He lived almost another year. (The president did not refer to the name of the products in his official communication, but Claude Gubler, Mitterrand's official doctor, later published a book entitled *Le Grand Secret* in which he revealed that the commotion regarding the president's treatment indeed concerned the Beljanski cancer-specific formulas.)

The Beljanski research team was left in peace by both the government and pharmaceutical industry as long as Mitterrand lived. It was usual for these two powerful institutions to work hand-in-hand against natural and nontoxic therapies.

In his last days, the ex-president maintained an office in Paris and was often spotted strolling along the Seine and browsing in bookstores. During this time, nobody bothered the Beljanskis, and the demand for the products increased considerably.

The files concerning the commercial market authorizations were nearing completion to be sent to the Health Ministry. The preparation of the documents had involved a lot of work for many years and enormous expenses. But now the formulas were about to receive the blessing of the French authorities. Everything seemed resolved.

Mitterrand succumbed to prostate cancer on January 8, 1996, after serving longer (14 years) as France's president than anyone since Napoleon III, leaving behind "a mixed legacy that is bound to fascinate and confound historians for decades to come," said *Time Paris* Bureau Chief Thomas Sancton.

In a climate full of jealousy, pettiness and rivalries, it was impossible for Mirko Beljanski to ever be acknowledged as a contributor to the welfare of humankind. The establishment could not accept that one totally independent scientist could be recognized for his discoveries. They decided to take harsh action by depriving him of the one thing that he needed: his laboratory, "because," as Monique declared, "they could no longer deny the truth in results that proved to be so efficacious."

At 6 a.m. on the morning of October 9, 1996, the GIGN, trained to deal with violence, riots, and terrorism, in what was clearly an over-the-top operation involving one helicopter and 80 antiterrorist soldiers, struck. Interestingly enough, the GIGN were not the police but a French Army Special-Forces Unit (this implies the order came from the highest levels of the government).

The GIGN, wearing flack vests, carrying machine guns and clubs, leading leashed police dogs, blowing whistles, padlocking entrance doors, and worse, closed down the Beljanskis' laboratory. Thus, the Beljanski lab was abruptly shut tight, and its salaried researchers locked out.

In an egregious abdication of their particular responsibility, members of the French media observed what was happening but remained silent. No effort was spared to humiliate Mirko or his research staff. But it was Mirko who was being martyred. The 73-year-old scientist was roused from bed, placed in handcuffs, and held for questioning for 24 hours with a bail set at an amount much higher than his entire retirement pension. He was not given information about his rights nor with what he was being charged. Monique was put under house arrest in Paris, unable to leave the premises or to use the phone to ask for legal aid or to know what was going on with her husband.

Again, before due process of law that would allow for charges and evidence and a chance to defend one's self—a fundamental human right—was allowed to take its course, the French Assistant Attorney General's Office issued an order recommending immediate destruction of all Beljanski products.

As for the AMM filing documentation, the police went to the offices of the special consultants who were putting the finishing touches on the market authorization files and took them all.

Of course, once the laboratory was ransacked, papers destroyed and samples taken, in his report No. 470/96, on August 7, 1997, the policeman Kentzinger observed: "It was advisable that the documents that were seized, as well as the documents relative to those experiments, as well as the letters from the sick persons be destroyed to avoid a repetition of events, but also to guarantee medical secrecy, and therefore respect the confidentiality of this information."

But what did they take away from the examination of the reports of the sick persons? Many thousands of them, divided between two associations (CIRIS and another patient group) claiming that the products developed by Beljanski (prescribed by doctors, most often in conjunction with traditional treatments) had eliminated their discomfort and the undesirable effects of the chemotherapy and radiation therapy treatments; they testified to a remission of their sickness, a number of them for several years. (In truth, the papers contained communications supplied exclusively by the sick, which are not at all bound by medical confidentiality.)

Next, the Beljanski products were ordered to be taken out of the homes of the people who were using them. The French authorities made their way from home to home using any information gleaned from doctors as to who was getting the capsules. They broke into homes, terrorizing ordinary citizens battling contentious illnesses, turning them into criminals. This marked an outrageous violation of basic human rights. The people would not have it. Confiscations occurred so that cancer patients were left without their support and unfortunately, some died so soon after their treatments were taken that the deaths can be argued to have occurred as a result of this basic violation—all occurring without any proceedings in a civil or criminal court.

All this happened without a chance for Mirko to defend his work. He was deprived of his basic right to confront his accusers. He was deprived of a basic human right to have a hearing before an impartial judge, and to confront his accuser (or accusers) and he was deprived of a basic human right as a result of the destruction of his laboratory with absolutely no due process. His passport was confiscated allegedly so that he would not be able to travel to another country where he would have the freedom to make a safe nontoxic approach and what the French government forbid its people to have.

By decree of bureaucracy, the biologist was forbidden from speaking publicly, from publishing his research, or from writing for the press.

After having their Beljanski capsules taken away, patients flocked in overflowing crowds to protest, demonstrating in the streets of Paris and Lyons while carrying signs demanding: "We want the Beljanski products!"

In Paris and Lyons, thousands of French citizens, including sick people in a panic from their fear of death, fighting to get their chosen treatments returned, took to the streets to protest. The following photo shows pro-Beljanski demonstrations involving thousands of French citizens on the streets of Paris and Lyons.

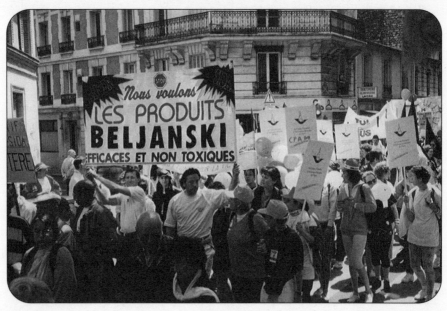

All of this ate away at the morale and health of Mirko, who could not live, in the literal sense of the word, through such injustice. One month after the raid on St. Prim, Mirko fell ill and soon was diagnosed with acute myeloid leukemia.

Day after day, nourished by the stress of the harassment he endured, Mirko's health dramatically worsened. He was no longer in possession of his own products and had to undergo standard chemotherapy. Throughout the proceedings, Mirko received several summonses to appear in court but, due to his hospitalization, could not. As a result, he and his family were hounded by notices demanding astronomical sums, millions of francs, without any justification, despite their constant appeals (even their financial file was not released to them). In addition, the French administration believed it necessary to freeze the Beljanski assets.

The illness that Mirko developed was very brutal. His products and his laboratory—his life work—had been taken away; his survival was in danger, and he was no longer interested in living.

During a short interval of remission, after undergoing two chemotherapy sessions, Mirko and his daughter Sylvie, by now an attorney living in New York City, organized the transfer of all information to be taken to America where they hoped medical freedom existed and his work could continue to inspire researchers.

Not long afterwards, it became clear that the hospital physicians would not be able to stop the progress of Mirko's disease. He thus decided to stop all transfusions and treatments and returned home to die.

In the meantime, ever practical and dedicated, he pored over his files and advised on all matters that he had extensively researched and studied. "He tried to put things in easy-to-understand language so that more people would have access," Sylvie said.

Hence, a highly professional long-playing video presentation of his work, based on interviews, was taped upon Sylvie's request in France shortly before his passing.

On the 28th of October 1998, Mirko died.

His burial was on October 30, 1998.

After Mirko's passing, Sylvie worked with Monique to file a legal action in the European Court of Human Rights against the Republic of France for the violation of fundamental human rights of a scientist to pursue his research.

On May 23, 2002, almost four years after his death, the European Court of Human Rights issued a decree in Strasbourg asserting that Mirko Beljanski had been denied a fair trial and the opportunity to defend his legacy and the scientific value of his research. The lower courts should have taken into account his age, state of health, and his right to due process. The European Court of Human Rights *unanimously* ruled that his right to be granted a fair trial in a reasonable time frame had been seriously violated.

France tried but never succeeded in destroying a man, an innovative researcher who asked for nothing except to contribute to humanity. He had chosen the country to become his own, naively believing in idealistic notions. But the flow of ideas and scientific concepts is harder to break than the life of one man.

Part II
America

CHAPTER EIGHT

The Columbia Connection

The United States of America was perhaps the only hope for the survival of Mirko's work, and New York City was, naturally, the hub of this hope. "To my family, America represented a country that gives everybody a chance based on the quality of one's contribution. America was also a beacon of hope during the dark years of the German occupation," said Sylvie. "Back in 1998, my father's health was rapidly failing. Even though I was coming from a very different background as a practicing French attorney, with no specific or formal scientific training, I felt a moral obligation to carry on his work. What I respect so much about the United States is that it is a far more liberal society in terms of allowing consumers access to a wide range of natural health products. "Therefore, knowing of the scientific documentation of my father's work, my first move was to meet with medical doctors who had been using my father's products for many years and who were, in fact, much more knowledgeable about them than I. I was then shocked and humbled by the way they were praising my father, his work, and the results they got with the products. Many qualified the results as 'unique.'"

The first U.S. symposium was held in 1999. French, Belgian and Israeli physicians flew to New York City to share their clinical experience with Beljanski's products with their American colleagues. In attendance was Michael B. Schachter, M.D., one of a growing number of physicians interested in what is now known in the United States as Complementary and Alternative Medicine or CAM.

Schachter had never heard the name "Beljanski" before, but when he got a personal call from an old friend, Patrick McGrady, Jr., who urged him to attend, saying he would learn some new things that may very well help his patients, he decided to go. Patrick McGrady, Jr., was a well-known author and researcher who offered an information service for cancer patients called CANHELP. McGrady passed away in 2003, and the service continues today under breast cancer survivor Madeleen Herreshoff.

Dr. Schachter sees more than 1,000 patients a year, enjoys a strong reputation for integrity, and uses a conservative yet integrative medical approach. In other words, he's got the credibility to be taken seriously. Schachter graduated *magna cum laude* from Columbia College in the City of New York. He earned his Medical Degree from Columbia University's College of Physicians and Surgeons in 1965. He received three years of psychiatric training at the Downstate Medical Center in Brooklyn, New York, and was board certified in psychiatry in 1971. He joins many other Columbia-based physicians and health experts who've embraced CAM.

In 1974, along with the late Dr. David Sheinkin, he established one of the first nutritionally oriented orthomolecular and holistic medical practices in New York State in Nyack. In 1991, Dr. Schachter moved his office to Suffern, New York, where it occupies 6,000 square feet, currently has 25 employees, and is known as the Schachter Center for Complementary Medicine.

Dr. Schachter has been extremely active in the field of alternative and complementary medicine. He served as vice-president of the Academy of Orthomolecular Psychiatry (AOP), president of the American College for Advancement in Medicine (ACAM) and has achieved the status of advanced proficiency in chelation therapy from this organization. He has also been president of the Foundation for the Advancement of Innovative Medicine (FAIM).

Dr. Schachter had worked extensively with cancer patients utilizing alternative therapies since 1975. He was familiar with a wide range of alternative therapeutic modalities and had incorporated several of them into his daily work with cancer patients. These have included dietary suggestions, intravenous infusions of vitamin C, enzyme therapy, amygdalin or laetrile therapy, various immune-enhancing methods, hydrazine sulfate, herbs, homeopathy, methods of detoxification, and psychosocial modalities, including visualization.

"The magnitude of Beljanski's findings struck me as being significant. They were so well-researched," said Schachter. "I've always felt the current paradigm only barely scratched the surface of our understanding of the true causes and most successful approaches to cancer. I was quite impressed with both the science presented in the lectures and the apparent benefits obtained by patients receiving the products. Following the conference, I spent a great deal of time reviewing the material and began to use these nutritional supplements with some of my cancer patients. Again, I was impressed with the results that many of the patients achieved with these nutritional supplements, as I incorporated them into my approach to supporting and managing cancer patients, using a wide variety of complementary and alternative approaches, sometimes with conventional treatment administered by surgeons, radiotherapists, and oncologists, and sometimes in place of these conventional approaches. As I was impressed with Dr. Beljanski's work, I decided to share this information, since his work is virtually unknown in the United States.

"To me, Dr. Beljanski has clearly made significant contributions to the understanding of carcinogenesis and has pioneered work that may be extremely beneficial to cancer patients. Modern medicine continues to struggle with helping patients who develop cancer and chronic viral diseases, such as hepatitis C and AIDS," Dr. Schachter said. "The most frequently used treatments for these conditions often have significant adverse effects and in many cases little potential benefits. Complementary and alternative practitioners constantly search for innovative ideas and products that may help their patients without causing side effects.

"During my entire professional life, I have devoted myself to learning about various health-enhancing programs and products to better understand health and disease and to help my patients. I am hungry to learn everything I can about what health and disease are all about. I regard it as my life's mission."

In 2002, Dr. Schachter made his own presentation about Beljanski's work at the American College for Advancement in Medicine in Washington, D.C., to American physicians, and he published a paper in the FAIM organization's *Innovation*, a non-peer-reviewed magazine.

Based on the clearly anecdotal but nonetheless suggestive evidence that Dr. Schachter accumulated in his medical practice, it was clear that patients using the Beljanski molecules were experiencing largely positive outcomes. While he hadn't conducted a formal study, Dr. Schachter was influencing other doctors and researchers who were open to the possibility that alternative medicine could help cancer patients. (I present Dr. Schachter in his own words, describing his patients' comprehensive CAM programs, in Appendix A.)

One of these people of influence was another Columbia University-based physician, Dr. Aaron Katz, a mainstream urologist with a reputation as one of New

York's leading prostate experts, according to *New York* magazine. He had recently been named as director of the Center for Holistic Urology at the university's Physicians and Surgeons Hospital where Dr. Schachter also trained.

"Initially, I learned about phytomedicines from my patients who were taking them for prostate conditions and using them for effectively lowering their PSAs," said Dr. Katz. "Like most physicians (who tend to be very conservative), I obviously started on a more traditional allopathic approach. When I started my academic practice at Columbia University, I was given an opportunity to work with Dr. Robert Atkins at the famous Atkins Center in Manhattan where they were educating patients about low-carb eating and using other holistic practices that are sometimes broadly referred to as alternative medicine.

"At the outpatient hospital, the physicians there saw patients all day long and they even had a pharmacy onsite. They didn't take any insurance, except Medicare. That was perhaps one reason why innovative findings were coming out of the Atkins Clinic. I would go there one day a week; they'd line up about 30 patients with prostate and urological problems, and I was the consultant. I worked there for four years from 1993 to 1997. While working there, I finished my residency and this very conservative medical training involving everything about oncology.

"Here I am working at Columbia University four days a week and I go there one day a week and see these people who are on herbs and nutrients, and at first I'm thinking to myself, 'This is a bunch of crap! What are you guys taking this for? It's not gonna work!'

"Yet as a doctor, you learn to listen to patients, if you are a good doctor. They were telling me things like, 'You know, I was on this medication, my doctor wanted me to have my prostate out, and instead I was taking this herb or that herb, and I'm doing fine.'

"And it wasn't just one patient; it was a lot of patients. So I said, 'You know what? Maybe there's something to this. Maybe this is real.'" He lobbied for the Center for Holistic Urology at Columbia University. "I was a little bit unsure of myself, because here I am this urologist opening up a holistic center, but I did have the support of my chairman, Dr. Carl Olson, who is a world-renowned urologic surgeon; he even terms himself a 'maximal invasive surgeon'—but he also felt that yes, maybe there was a role for this aspect of complementary medicine, and that maybe I could obtain funding to examine the herbal compounds and nutrition and so forth.

"So the mainstream wasn't as closed as one might think, at least not at Columbia, and we all did see the benefit of it. And then in my practice at Columbia, I thought, maybe this is a niche for me. Because everybody at my department was like, 'If we see any patients that want that herbal crap, we're going to send them to Aaron.' Or, 'We saw Mr. Jones, and he wants some of that herbal stuff; we told him to go see Dr. Katz. We don't know anything about that.' These guys are traditionally trained surgeons, and how do they make their money? By operating. If it's a big operation, they get big money…and it's not to say they don't cure patients with surgery, because they do. And I'm not saying that there's no role for surgery in certain patients, because I do a lot of surgeries. But I also know that we overtreat, in terms of prostate cancer, way too many cancers in this country with overly aggressive therapies that leave men, unfortunately, with significant side effects: impotence and incontinence. And unfortunately no therapy, even surgery, is 100 percent effective all the time."

Could Mirko's work help men with one of the most common cancers, that of the prostate? Prostate cancer is the second most common cause of cancer death among men worldwide, in particular throughout Europe and the United States. When prostatic tissue is examined microscopically, cancer is found in 50 percent of males over age 70 and in virtually all males over age 90. Most of the time, such cancers never cause symptoms, but 3 percent of men exhibiting diseased prostate tissue changes die of the malignancy.

In fact, many men with prostate cancer now know it is probably not invasive and that they will die of other causes long before it ever spreads. Thus, extreme treatment isn't always the right way to go.

"Most doctors today do not know much about holistic urology. I am one of the few urologists involved in clinical and laboratory studies of natural formulas, so I see firsthand the best and truly worst from both sides," said Dr. Katz. "I simply want to give men everywhere the best information about integrative prostate health because the integrative health system is the greatest and most beneficial to men. My uniquely positioned work at Columbia and the Center for Holistic Urology allows me more time than probably anyone in America today to study holistic urology.

"So it is my sincere desire to help all men everywhere to attain good health with the best of all disciplines—a balanced, successful approach to maintaining or regaining and then maintaining your health."

Dr. Katz met with Beljanski's daughter and widow who provided him with the background and explained Mirko's lifelong interest in plants and treatments devoid of toxicity.

"I asked Sylvie a lot of questions about her father," he recalled. The two discussed her father's work during several meetings in New York City. She shared with Dr. Katz her father's many peer-reviewed scientific articles and research results, especially his applied research after leaving the Pasteur Institute and the Pharmaceutical Faculty.

Dr. Katz recalls, "I brought home a lot of reading material!" Bringing fresh eyes to Dr. Beljanski's research seemed to work. "I thought his science was excellent and definitely many decades ahead of his time. He was definitely the first to open up the whole field of structural DNA, and in this alone his vision of the secrets of life was wholly unique and powerful.

"The next step was to take Beljanski's body of work and study it using rigorous scientific procedures." Everything had to be repeated, he told Sylvie. American doctors would want to see data from American labs.

All of Beljanski's work would have to be repeated and reconfirmed in America for it to be accepted by the mainstream—and it would need to be extended into clinical trials. The first step was to retest and confirm Mirko's basic findings pertaining to certain plant extracts in the Columbia University center's laboratory.

Dr. Katz and the scientific team in his department started from the very beginning with cells in cultures, and then grafted mice with cancer cells. Their research paid off big time with a notable peer-reviewed article in the November 2006 (29; 1065-73) issue of the *International Journal of Oncology* that was titled, "Antiprostate Cancer Activity of a Beta-Carboline Alkaloid Enriched Extract from *Rauwolfia vomitoria*." Debra L. Bemis, Ph.D., and other top researchers from the Department of Urology, College of Physicians and Surgeons, Columbia University Medical Center and the Center for Holistic Urology reported on the antiprostate cancer activity of this extract *in vitro* and *in vivo*.[17]

Rauwolfia vomitoria extract standardized for beta-carboline alkaloids was tested for its ability to influence the growth and survival of the human LNCaP prostate cancer cell line that was developed to study how well substances cause or prevent cell proliferation.

Among the Columbia University team's findings were the following:

"In mice, the cancerous prostate LNCaP cells were treated with the extract or placebo, and tumor growth was measured for 5 weeks. The effects of the extract were measured on cell proliferation and apoptosis, the latter is a form of healthy programmed cell death that causes malfunctioning cells to destroy themselves before they invade other tissues.

"Rauwolfia extract decreased *in vitro* cell growth in a dose-dependent manner… demonstrated that apoptosis [programmed cell death, a good thing where immortal cancer cells are involved] was induced only at the highest concentration tested (500 microg/ml). Tumor volumes were decreased by 60 percent, 70 percent and 58 percent in the groups fed the 75, 37.5, or 7.5 mg/kg Rauwolfia, respectively. The *Rauwolfia vomitoria* extract significantly suppressed the growth and cell cycle progression of LNCaP cells, *in vitro* and *in vivo*."

In other words, the extract was significantly interfering with the progression of cancer, much as Beljanski's own research had shown. Dr. Katz had done one of the most important things in science: He had independently confirmed another researcher's findings.

Indeed, Dr. Bemis, the primary researcher, went further and stated in an interview with the author, "Our studies thus far indicate that both the Rauwolfia and Pao extracts suppress prostate tumor cell growth in culture and *in vitro* and also *in vivo*, but it appears to accomplish this effect through different mechanisms which we studied accurately. Our data from the Pao pereira studies is now in the process of being published." The fact that the plant extracts kill the cancerous cells through two different mechanisms suggests that combined, they could have a more powerful anticancer effect.

"We found there was real scientific evidence that the combination of *Rauwolfia vomitoria* and Pao pereira had a powerful inhibitory effect on the ability of prostate cells to grow and divide. That was very interesting to our team," said Katz.

The Columbia team's preclinical findings were again published in the Spring 2009 issue of the *Journal of the Society of Integrative Oncology*.[18] Dr. Bemis and co-researchers from the Center for Holistic Urology reported that, "Bark extracts from the Amazonian rainforest tree *Geissospermum vellosii* (Pao pereira), enriched in beta-carboline alkaloids have significant anticancer activities in certain preclinical models. Because of the predominance of prostate cancer as a cause of cancer-related morbidity and mortality for men of Western countries, we preclinically tested the *in vitro* and *in vivo* effects of a Pao pereira extract against a prototypical human prostate cancer cell line, LNCaP. When added to cultured LNCaP cells, Pao pereira extract significantly suppressed cell growth in a dose-dependent fashion and induced apoptosis."

A clinical trial began in 2006 and enrolled some 42 patients with elevated prostate specific antigen (PSA) readings (averaging 8 to 10 on the PSA scale) and a negative biopsy—a group of men that in the industrialized world numbers in the millions.

These men have ticking time bombs in their prostates: They have elevated PSAs, but they don't have cancer. In some cases, urologists prescribe powerful drugs to their patients that have a number of side effects (depressed sexual libido, impotence, gynecomastia, and the potential for birth defects). In a world where medicine would be unbiased by profits, these drugs would not be considered a big hit because of these side effects. But this is what men nationwide are getting because it is one of the only options out there for men. And the idea for many men and their doctors of simply doing nothing ("watchful waiting") isn't an appealing alternative, either.

"If you look at some of the clinical trials with men who have had a biopsy based on their PSAs—even men with PSAs of around 2 to 2.5 still have a 25 percent incidence of cancer. As you go above PSA readings of 10, some 70 percent of men are likely to develop cancer," said Dr. Katz in a series of articles and interviews conducted by a reporter at *The Doctors' Prescription for Healthy Living* magazine in 2007 and 2009.

One of the primary goals of the clinical trial was to determine if the plant extracts were safe. The research team did a dose-escalation trial. The trial started at two capsules but has gone much higher, and so far all doses tested have been without side effects. In addition to this clinical trial, Dr. Katz is following patients to look at quality-of-life issues and how the formula affects urinary function. What do we know so far?

"As our researchers crunch numbers and prepare our publications, I think there are some things we can safely say that we are seeing and that we can speak about generally. We now know that this combination of Beljanski's extracts can significantly lower PSAs in a 12-month period. Also, we have had very few patients convert to prostate cancer and have found a number of patients who have had a dramatic improvement in their urinary symptoms. Men are clearly having less frequency, better streams, and better flow rates. They are not getting up at night as often.

"All of this quite apparent improvement in their urinary flow and prostate health has been an interesting finding for us. We simply did not expect to see so much help for enlarged prostates (since we're also examining the ability of the extracts to interact with cells at the DNA level). I am very encouraged. We have even been going up to eight pills a day without adverse events. Nobody has dropped out of the trial from side effects, either, which shows a lot, since you almost always have a few dropouts even on placebo.

"The bottom line is that it appears our early results are reason to be very encouraged by Beljanski's extracts' ability to lower PSA and help older men urinate better, too. In some way, we now realize, the results may be better than saw palmetto (an herb generally accepted as proven for men's health), although we can't say for sure because we have not tested Rauwolfia and Pao pereira against saw palmetto. Sure, we would love to do side by side comparisons with saw palmetto and Finasteride. Obviously, I'd like to extend our clinical trial as well," said Dr. Katz.

So how important are Beljanski's findings to men's health? "There are a lot of men undergoing PSA screenings," Dr. Katz said. "The PSA supposedly stands for prostate specific antigen, but I say it is more accurately, 'patient stimulated anxiety.' When men's PSA is elevated, there could be many reasons for this, having nothing to do with cancer. One of the more common reasons is that the prostate has grown in a benign fashion. The more prostate cells you have, the more PSA gets into your bloodstream. Still, because we don't know if it's benign or malignant, many men undergo a prostate biopsy to make sure they do not have prostate cancer. If it is negative, just benign growth, then doctors might prescribe finasteride or not do anything. But what we know now is that these cells that are growing can develop into cancer, and we would like to stop them from growing into cancer. Also, if the cells keep growing even in benign fashion, they will grow around the urethra and push in on it and provoke urinary symptoms in men. Many men in their 60s and 70s have this problem where their growth is benign but their stream is weak, and they are getting up at night and don't urinate as well. That's where we want to lower the growth and division of prostate cells—and that's what we think we have shown with the extracts. That's why we do these trials: to learn about medicine. After all, Viagra's use for erectile dysfunction was discovered after researchers were initially looking at lung conditions in men. We want to gather our data in a scientific system and sit back and look at the results and offer rational explanations and find the best way to use these tools in the interest of men's health."

Although American urologists have sometimes been reluctant to take the European studies as seriously as those published in U.S. medical journals, thanks to the pioneering work of Dr. Katz, Mirko's work is gaining acceptance among medical colleagues—and increasingly, doctors are becoming interested in how to integrate these natural remedies into their patients' health plans.

"We don't get any antagonism when we're working with our projects," said Dr. Katz. "What we're doing here at the Center for Holistic Urology at Columbia University is saying to people there may be a role for these compounds and we are going to test them, and we are going to put them through tough clinical testing, much as if they were a pharmaceutical and see if they pass muster and see if they have a mechanism of action. Rather than just handing them out to patients, we are doing appropriate scientific investigations and testing them out in the laboratory and seeing how they work with the patients, and if you do that and if you run it through university settings, then you might be open to some criticism but much less. What we're seeing is helping patients.

"Dr. Beljanski's fundamental vision is beginning to pay off in the way so many hoped for in his own lifetime. This compound has all of the molecular and biochemical studies showing why it works; how it actually recognizes the three-dimensional structure through the laddering and bonding of DNA. He really did get it right. This is something that has great potential to help patients."

CHAPTER NINE

Breakthrough Research

At the same time that Mirko was being forced out of the Pasteur Institute, a young doctoral student from America was arriving there on a research scholarship. Although he didn't personally meet Mirko at that time, he remembered that people talked about him; that people respected his work and how he was able to survive at the Institute.

"In those days the Pasteur Institute was the leading institute of molecular biology in the non-English-speaking world," said James Grutsch, Ph.D. Dr. Grutsch is the clinical trial consultant to the prestigious Cancer Treatment Centers of America, a network of regional hospitals throughout the United States, dedicated to fighting cancer with the very latest and most successful integrative tools from both conventional and complementary medicine.

"But from what I was able to glean, Beljanski's view of DNA came into direct conflict with that of Jacques Monod, the director of the Institute, who claimed DNA to be the only omnipotent molecule. Monod even then had a reputation as a tyrant."

Everybody knew. "The French researchers were very driven, worked very hard, and were very competitive in those days," Dr. Grutsch said. "I read Mirko Beljanski's work though, and I thought about it. He was right on target, and if he survived all those years under a director like Monod, then he must have been a fine scientist. He was a darn good scientist and he had done all of the work to show us that we could actually save lives with a certain type of RNA fragment."

So when Dr. Grutsch began to learn about the fragments for the first time, he had, so to speak, been primed himself by his own early educational experience in Paris. As mentioned, platelets are blood cell fragments formed from megakary-

ocytes necessary for normal blood clotting; without them, the body has no secondary mechanism to prevent internal bleeding: they halt the leakage of red blood
cells from an injured blood vessel. By design, platelets are not long lived in the
body and usually are around only nine days, so your body must constantly reman-
ufacture its platelets to replace those it loses. When people undergo chemotherapy or radiotherapy for cancer treatment, these platelets are destroyed. But why
are platelet levels such a problem for cancer patients?

The normal blood platelet count ranges from 150,000 to 450,000 for every
milliliter of blood for a healthy individual. However, radiotherapy and chemotherapy attack not only cancer cells but also the body's healthy bone marrow, gas-
trointestinal tract, and mouth. The bone marrow is where new blood cells are synthesized, and if the levels of platelets become too low, as they frequently do during chemotherapy or radiotherapy, all treatment must be stopped.

Thrombocytopenia is when platelets are lost from the bloodstream faster than
they can be replaced. "The result is that, all of a sudden, you get incredibly low levels of both white blood cells, for which we have some drugs now, and platelets, for
which we can't do anything other than transfusions and wait," said Dr. Grutsch.

Although the pharmaceutical industry has come up with drugs that are able to
help the body maintain white blood cell counts, the same is not so for the platelets
responsible for blood clotting. Many chemotherapy and radiotherapy protocols,
which might otherwise have saved the lives of cancer patients, are halted at least
temporarily because of dangerously low platelet counts, Dr. Grutsch explained.
"It's a major problem in cancer treatment."

At the Cancer Treatment Centers of America, the oncologists and medical
experts are constantly seeking out new ways to help patients fight back against
cancer and support their health through chemotherapy and radiotherapy.

Nearly three decades after leaving Paris, Dr. Grutsch looked at the results that
the patients' association in France had collected as well as dossiers of toxicology
created by many experts to confirm the nontoxicity of the RNA fragments.
Together with oncologists Robert Levin and Mary Ann Daehler, the team began
recruiting patients from the CTCA population to receive the RNA fragments.
These were some of the most difficult cases, patients who simply could not complete their chemotherapy regimens, due to low platelet counts. By June 2007, Dr.
Grutsch was crunching data, and it was looking good for the approximately 70
patients who had participated in the study.

Beljanski was right after all—the RNA fragments were boosting the bone marrow DNA replication, rejuvenating the stem cells, and increasing the number of platelets. Beljanski's RNA fragments "were clearly helping the patients to maintain their platelet counts," he said. "There was no way around the outcome. This product was helping our patients in a meaningful way to get through their chemotherapy. These patients had developed terminal cancers but in the absence of RNA fragments, they had failed several rounds of chemotherapy—we had some patients with 10 or 11 uncompleted cycles—who were finally getting through all of their rounds. With higher doses of RNA fragments, they were going into recovery numbers and they could continue their treatments. They had all sorts of cancer—breast, pancreatic, colon, and lung. What they had in common was their particularly challenging chemotherapies—with incredible failure rates. These were very challenging patients who had failed nine or 10 earlier rounds."

This is such an important finding that Dr. Grutsch said the CTCA is anxious to begin enrolling patients in a larger randomized clinical trial.

"Our next step is going to be to do a randomized clinical trial," he told the authors. "I think we are going to do some really important clinical trials now. It is urgent to help our patients and cancer patients everywhere, obviously. You really want to treat these people in a timely fashion, twice a month, and you could probably increase cure rates by a significant level, so potentially, this could be very, very important, and we want to be the first to discover it," he emphasized.

How difficult will it be to recruit patients? "Once our oncologists realize that these specific RNA fragments potentially work, they will be very good at recruiting all the patients we need; recruiting patients will not be an issue. You have to believe that the product has a real likelihood of working based on our first clinical trial. We are getting real experience with this product and feel really comfortable with it. But we have to keep going with more clinical trials, because oncologists like lots of data points. The things they do are challenging, just keeping patients alive from treatment cycle to treatment cycle. They like to know what they have to work with."

Dr. Grutsch, nearly three decades removed from his blissful early days at the Pasteur Institute, has all the enthusiasm of the young scientist who thinks he can leave his mark on the scientific world.

"I have to tell you something," he said. "I have been doing clinical studies for 20 years—but this trial is definitely my favorite. I think this one has the greatest potential by far to have the most impact."

"I think of Beljanski's RNA fragments as food," said Dr. Grutsch, "This product is food because these RNA fragments can be thought of as essential nutrients. I know most people don't realize this. They're not up on the latest nutritional information. Every time you eat salads or meat, you are eating RNA, so your diet already has a large quantity of RNAs. Intact RNAs do not behave as RNA fragments, though, so think of Beljanski's RNA fragments as super RNA. You get patients who are stressed, and if you give them RNA fragments, they actually maintain healthy platelet counts. We've tried other very similarly conceived ideas from other sources proclaiming to do the same thing and they did not do it. There is something about what Beljanski specifically uncovered that is completely unique because of their specificity.

"One of the biggest innovations is that the Food and Drug Administration now requires baby formula manufacturers to put in long- and short-chain RNAs in their products, so babies have less rounds of diarrhea. RNAs seem to be essential nutrients, especially if your body is under incredible physiological stress. But this information was really only discovered in the past 10 to 15 years, and again Beljanski provided so much of the research findings first and most accurately."

Indeed RNAs are good for overall health but only these specific RNA fragments work on immunity. Today, the data are overwhelming. Dr. Beljanski discovered in the course of his research many different biological roles for a variety of small RNAs, but only RNA fragments act as primers for DNA bone marrow. It was very interesting to compare two sorts of RNA fragments: the one that Beljanski prepared (from RNA isolated from E. coli K12, a bacteria which is a natural species from the human intestinal tract and recognized by the National Institutes of Health as a totally innocuous strain) and common RNA fragments made from yeast RNA.

Clearly, from the results that Dr. Grutsch obtained, Mirko's very specific fragments were able to stimulate healthy platelet levels.

Again, we have an independent confirmation of the work. This discovery has the potential to help many tens of thousands of cancer patients every year in the United States alone. The RNA fragments have proven to be safe and nontoxic.

Besides the initial step of cell division, which is the result of the selectivity, there is no other intervention of these RNA fragments. These RNA fragments do not interfere with other cells. They simply support the body's ability to naturally enhance the generation of white blood cells and platelets. They have been conceived on the model that, very probably, nature itself uses to promote the renewal of its cells. But, then, to peer into the secrets of nature was Beljanski's ultimate genius.

CHAPTER TEN

Taking Charge
of Your Health

CANCER PREVENTION & THE ENVIRONMENT

In an era when pollution is extreme, regulations and screening of chemicals for toxicity should be an absolute requisite. In this regard, the Beljanski test for detecting destabilizing compounds, (i.e., pro-carcinogens) is revolutionary—and it is a science that promises to yield real progress in the strategy that has been called the key to winning the war against cancer: "prevention." Senator Arlen Spector of Pennsylvania has put forward legislation consistently raising the budget for NCI and directing that money toward prevention. Prevention as a concept is most important. But who can imagine prevention with toxic chemical drugs? Prevention requires natural, non-harmful means that may be used regularly by people who are still healthy. It is not, then, a question of a drug that can be toxic or disturb their physiological state. As the first green molecular biologist, Mirko was conscious that natural phytochemicals that are active and nontoxic (which is not always the case), know how to behave in a biological environment, and thus are well-tolerated. Mirko always wanted to give priority to such molecules and put them in the place they deserved to be. He was not "green" because it was fashionable, but for scientific, biological, and moral reasons with strong arguments to support the evolution of his science.

A limited number of groups determine whether substances are carcinogens—among these, the federal Environmental Protection Agency, the National Toxicology Program, within the U.S. Department of Health and Human Services (DHHS), and the International Agency for Research on Cancer (IARC), run by the World Health Organization (WHO). [Note: also, in California, the California Environmental Protection Agency, Office of Environmental Health Hazard Assessment, pursuant to the Safe Drinking Water and Toxic Enforcement Act of 1986 (Proposition 65).] Such groups review the latest in scientific evidence and make a determination whether a chemical causes cancer or not. Sometimes there isn't enough evidence to make a ruling. Though the organizations examine many of the same chemicals, they don't always agree. Even when a chemical is recognized as a carcinogen, it may be allowed to be in commerce, as in the case of 1,4-dioxane in children's bubble baths and shampoos. For example, on January 1, 1988, California, under Proposition 65, listed 1,4-dioxane as a chemical known to cause cancer, which means that products containing the chemical must bear a warning statement if sold in California.

Even when compounds are screened, our past technology has offered clearly unsatisfactory results. The Ames test is a screening test that is used to help identify chemicals that affect the nucleic acids of DNA. The test exposes Salmonella bacteria to chemicals and looks for changes in the requirements for amino acids in order to grow. These changes result from mutations that occur when the coding sequence of DNA is altered in certain locations. Many chemicals that cause mutations can cause cancer in animals or in people. But over time, the test was found to be a less reliable predictor of carcinogenesis than had been hoped. Some chemicals that are known to cause cancer do not test positive in the Ames test, and some chemicals that test positive do not cause cancer. In addition, many chemicals that cause cancer do not cause mutations. Nonetheless, the test is still considered an important part of assessing the safety of new chemicals.

A series of published studies shows that Beljanski's tests for procarcinogens could be far more productive in preventing cancer. These studies challenge a basic premise in cancer research—that cancer is produced for the most part by genes that have undergone mutation.

In the field of prevention, Beljanski's pioneering work has been vindicated by Dr. Donald Malins who presented his findings in the prestigious *Proceedings of the National Academy of Science* showing that cancer is not so much the product of dysfunctional genes as it is the result of widespread DNA structural damage caused by a class of highly reactive chemicals known as "free radicals," produced in response to metabolic and environmental stress.

Malins performed his work while with the Biochemical Oncology Program, Pacific Northwest Research Institute in Seattle. In the April 2004 issue of *Environmental Health Perspectives*, Malins published "Structural Changes in Gill DNA Reveal the Effects of Contaminants on Puget Sound Fish."

Chemical markers of sediment contamination [e.g., polynuclear aromatic hydro-carbons (PAHs) and polychlorinated biphenyls (PCBs)] were established. "Marked structural damage was found in the gill DNA of the DR fish," his team wrote. "The evidence implies that environmental chemicals contribute to the DNA changes in the gill. The damaged DNA is a promising marker for identifying, through gill biop-sies, contaminant effects on fish." He co-authored another paper entitled, "Cancer-related Changes in Prostate DNA as Men Age and Early Identification of Metastasis in Primary Prostate Tumors." In this article in the April 29, 2003, issue of the *Proceedings of the National Academy of Sciences* (100; 9:5401-05) Malins noted, "This cancer-like phenotype, which was not found in the younger men (age [16 to 36]), appears to arise from progressive age-related damage to DNA. Strikingly, we were additionally able to discriminate between the DNA of primary prostate tumors and the DNA of primary prostate tumors from which distant metastases had been iden-tified. Moreover, logistic regression analysis was able to predict the probability that a tumor had metastasized with approximately 90 percent sensitivity and specificity. Collectively, these findings are particularly promising for identifying men at risk for developing prostate cancer, as well as for the early determination of whether a pri-mary tumor has progressed to the metastatic state."

Malins' several articles perfectly vindicate the Beljanski concept about the first steps toward cancer occurring, little by little, in the DNA, until a certain thresh-old, where this fundamental molecule evolves into a state that no longer allows for normal cell synthesis and physiological control—and we now know that he was right! Beljanski emphasized that DNA destabilization (Malins called it "disor-der") is progressive and cumulative. The effect of low levels of destabilization has a compounding effect that induces molecules to multiply over and over.

The March 22, 2004, issue of Fortune has an excellent article that asserts *there* has been no real progress in the treatment of the most common forms of cancer. Entitled "War on Cancer: Why the New Drugs Disappoint," the article cites NCI data showing that U.S. cancer mortality rates have increased and age-adjusted cancer mortality rates in response to treatment have not improved in several decades, despite the introduction of many new drugs.

On November 26, 2008, a report compiled by NCI, American Cancer Society, Centers for Disease Control and Prevention, and the North American Association of Central Cancer Registries and published online in the *Journal of the National Cancer Institute* found the first notable drop in incidence. Yet the decline was boosted by California, largely because of a comprehensive ban on smoking. It was the only state to show declines in both incidence and deaths from lung cancer in women. "It's a testament to the change in the lifestyle of the people of California," said Dr. Robert Figlin of the City of Hope Comprehensive Cancer Center in Duarte, California, in an article in *The Los Angeles Times*. However, the article cautioned that the declines may be temporary. Figlin added, "Baby boomers are reaching the age at which they develop cancer…so we should not be surprised if it changes direction again."

We have some sobering questions to ask. If we know that rates have leveled off in response to better prevention and diagnostic programs, why don't we continue to emphasize additional methods of prevention?

By scientific necessity, methods such as Beljanski's Oncotest should be examined. Cellular assaults on DNA can be measured before or even in the absence of mutations. Isn't this a more meaningful measure of toxicity?

People with cancer need help now. Massive funding shifts are in order. It is time for NCI to put an even greater emphasis on prevention and the use of selective molecules.

More than half of all cancer patients now embrace CAM as a method of prevention and health support. Most do not think of these as cures by any means but as part of a larger program that involves all aspects of health.

Unfortunately, there is a "cancer investigator" culture within NCI. Some have labeled NCI a "dysfunctional 'cancer culture'" as noted in the article in *Fortune*—victim of "a groupthink that pushes tens of thousands of physicians and scientists toward the goal of finding the tiniest improvements in treatment rather than genuine breakthroughs; that…rewards academic achievement and publication over all else."

Many cancer drugs have terrible side effects and often are no more effective than their older counterparts. In addition, they cost five times more. An article in the August 3, 2002, *British Medical Journal* (325;7358:269-271) from two Italian pharmacologists provided an overview of trials involving 12 new anticancer drugs that had been approved for the European market from 1995 to 2000. The researchers also compared these new drugs with older less-expensive therapies. No more greater rates of survival, quality of life or safety were found. "All of them, though, were several times more expensive than the old drugs. In one case, the price was 350 times higher."

How are we going to win the war against cancer if we aren't even trying to win?

Dr. Schachter in his Own Words

Among the most important decisions a cancer patient must make—in consultation with his physician or other health care practitioner—is whether to use conventional cancer treatments, which may include surgery, radiation, chemotherapy, antihormonal therapy or some of the newer monoclonal antibody treatments that target certain steps in the cancer process.

After evaluating the options, the patient must decide which treatments to undergo. More and more frequently, patients are discussing with their physician how these allopathic treatments can be supported by alternative approaches to promote health and wellness, while combating disease.

Under certain circumstances, after a careful evaluation of the risks and benefits of the specific conventional treatments being offered, the patient might decide that the benefits do not clearly outweigh the risks, and he or she might decide to forego the conventional treatments, instead focusing energy on an intensive, potentially less-toxic alternative approach.

The decision is complex and personal and requires the evaluation of many different factors relating to the person's disease and personal and cultural factors. This decision should only be made in the context of the physician-patient relationship. In some cases, patients will decide not to use any chemotherapy or radiotherapy. When I discuss the pros and cons of these treatments, I point out that the purpose of using radiation or chemotherapy is to kill cancer cells. Unfortunately, both radiation and chemotherapy have negative qualities, which I also discuss.

In fact, these treatments have four negative characteristics in common: (1) radiation and chemotherapy are mutagenic, which means that they cause mutations, and mutations in certain classes of genes relate to the development of cancer (for example mutations in proto-oncogenes result in oncogenes and accelerated cancer-cell growth, and mutations in tumor suppressor genes result in the brakes that control the cellular growth failing, so that cancer cells can grow out of control); (2) they are both carcinogenic, which means both of them are capable of causing secondary cancers, and, indeed, their use is well-known to increase the risk of developing secondary cancers after the initial treatment; (3) both of them are immune suppressive, which means they weaken one of the body's own mechanisms of controlling cancer cell growth by damaging natural killer cells and other immune functions; and finally, (4) they each have acute and chronic adverse side effects, depending on which treatments are used.

So, we commonly see loss of appetite, weight loss, diarrhea, pain, loss of hair, loss of red blood cells (anemia), low white blood cells, low platelets, neurological problems (pain or numbness in the extremities), fibrosis leading to impaired lung function, and many others. Many chronic, long-term effects of these treatments have not really been fully evaluated.

Conventional medicine has come up with a few articles recently suggesting that physicians need to become more aware of the inherent dangers in using diagnostic radiation. For example, a CT scan may expose a person to 100 times more radiation than a chest X-ray. Radiation exposure is cumulative, and one's lifetime exposure to radiation increases the risk of cancer, heart disease, and a variety other medical problems. Even a mammography increases one's risk of developing breast cancer and it is believed that two mammography pictures of a breast may increase the risk of breast cancer by 1 percent. Over time, this cumulative exposure quickly adds up.

Therapeutic radiotherapy for breast cancer exposes the patient to a much higher dose of radiation. A breast cancer patient may receive 3,000 RADs over several weeks. This is routine for women who have had a lumpectomy. The cost of the treatment is approximately $45,000. But, there is little or no evidence that this procedure improves overall survival. The only benefit may be a reduced risk of local recurrence. Most breast cancer patients are not aware of these facts, and when confronted with the information may opt for not doing radiation following their lumpectomy. They instead may decide to undergo an intensive health-enhancing alternative program that has no effect on or nourishes normal cells.

Another example in which the current recommended treatments may turn out not to be in the best interests of the patient is the treatment of prostate cancer. At the present time, men are usually screened with a blood test called the Prostate Specific Antigen or PSA. If it is slightly elevated or has increased significantly in the past year, the patient is referred to an urologist. Most often the urologist will recommend a prostate biopsy. What is ignored is the possibility that the very act of taking the prostate biopsy (often 12 or more snips of the prostate gland) may actually set up an inflammatory process that may contribute to prostatitis or even to the development of cancer.

If cancer is present, the possibility of increasing its spread as a result of the biopsy is ignored. The cancer patient is usually given three options, which are the following: (1) a radical prostatectomy; (2) radiation (either as external-beam radiation or the implantation of radioactive seeds); or (3) drugs that result in androgen deprivation. Each of these treatments is associated with significant short- and long-term adverse effects, such as problems with urination, problems with sexual functioning, and many others. What's more, careful evaluation of long-term survival statistics fails to show a clear-cut survival advantage with the localized prostate cancer treatments and the androgen-deprivation therapy."

The prostate cancer issue was recently demonstrated to me loud and clear. About three years ago, I met with a gentleman in his 70s who had recently been diagnosed with prostate cancer (Gleason Score 6, indicating a moderately aggressive prostate cancer). His PSA was about 10 (normal is below 4, so this was a significant elevation). His urologist strongly recommended radiation therapy and told him he would be dead in 18 months if he did not accept this recommendation.

This patient, whom I will call John, was still working full-time and managing an auto dealership. When he visited with me, he indicated that he did not want to do radiation therapy and wondered if he might manage his prostate cancer with alternative therapies. We set up a program involving changes in lifestyle that involved a fairly strict diet, intravenous vitamin C drips, some of the Beljanski products, and a number of other supplements. We also agreed to monitor him with physical examinations, PSA blood tests, and Power Doppler ultrasound of his prostate.

During the past three years, he has lost about 40 pounds (he was obese when he started) and has followed his program. As of this writing, there is no evidence that his cancer has worsened. His PSA has remained the same, and his Power Doppler has remained the same or has improved. He says he has never felt better.

About two years after I first saw John, he asked me if I would consult with his boss, Al, who was diagnosed with prostate cancer around the same time that John was diagnosed by the same urologist. Al was about the same age, and his clinical picture was very similar at the time of diagnosis. He also had a Gleason Score 6, had an elevated PSA, and was overweight. The same urologist recommended radiation for Al, and he decided to do it.

By the time I saw Al, the prostate cancer had spread. I offered him a complementary program. At first, he showed some interest, but then decided not to do this and instead just followed the advice of his urologist and oncologist. Several months later, John told me that Al was now considered terminal.

Although we have here only two cases, this story certainly suggests that for many men with prostate cancer, an intensive alternative program under a doctor's supervision might not only help control the prostate cancer, but might improve health in general. This story also suggests that following conventional advice for prostate cancer may not be beneficial for all who do so.

Yet, in some cases, we need the conventional methods. For example, if a person comes to me with a diagnosis of colon cancer that was diagnosed by a colonoscopy and wants to avoid surgery and instead do an intensive alternative program, I will strongly recommend surgery followed by the alternative program. In the case of colon cancer with no evidence of spread to vital organs, I believe surgery can be lifesaving and should be done. In the case of colon cancer, conventional therapy should be done because the survival statistics clearly show that it should.

On the other hand, I am not strongly impressed with the other conventional treatments that are often recommended with surgery. These may include radiation and chemotherapy. We have several long-term survivors with colon cancer who have not done chemotherapy, even though there may have been some lymph node involvement at the time of surgery. I believe every case must be evaluated on its own merits from many different perspectives.

At the Schachter Center for Complementary Medicine (in Rockland County, New York), some patients choose conventional treatment and others forgo it. Increasingly, patients with all types of cancer in various stages are showing a keen interest in complementary medicine, and surprisingly large numbers of patients actually choose to forgo conventional treatments completely.

The power of integrative medicine, also called CAM (Complementary Alternative Medicine), to enhance healing is relevant to both types of patients. Certainly, those who opt exclusively for the complementary or alternative or naturopathic modalities alone are aware that this approach can be very powerful. But CAM modalities are also extremely important for patients who decide to use conventional treatments as well. CAM is extraordinarily important for enhancing healing, supporting immune health, enhancing the positive effects of conventional treatments, and reducing adverse side effects.

I find my patients who use conventional treatment do well when they combine other alternative methods of support, ranging from nutrition, nutritional supplements, intravenous nutritional infusions, stress management (including meditation), exercise, and energy treatments, such as acupuncture.

At the Schachter Center, we make extensive use of the Beljanski formulas. These are used mostly in conjunction with dietary recommendations (such as avoiding sugar, alcohol, tobacco, chemicals added to food and many others), other nutritional supplements, infusions of selective nontoxic biological supplements like high-dose vitamin C, acupuncture, stress management, and an exercise program.

We always face challenges in the CAM field, as we are not well-funded like the doctors who work with the big-money drugs from Big Pharma. We know that we must always attempt to meet the challenges we face and not overstate our knowledge. According to our model, we use nutritional support and other modalities to improve normal physiological functions to encourage the body to heal itself. With this approach, it is often impossible to determine which of the various products or treatment modalities is responsible for most of the healing. In general, the supplements and other modalities work as a team and are synergistic. Nevertheless, I think the Beljanski products have been helpful for the majority of patients who have used them.

I have used the formulas with hundreds of patients since the year 2000. My impression is that they are very helpful. And this has been further borne out by the important experimental and clinical research being done on the combination of Pao pereira and *Rauwolfia vomitoria* by Aaron Katz, M.D., and Debra Bemis, Ph.D., of the Center for Holistic Urology at Columbia University, where the formula appears to be working effectively to support prostate health. What this means is that our very best medical scientists have compiled evidence that the formula is nontoxic, selective, and has real benefits.

Looking at the
Secrets of Life

Escalating cancer incidence with only modest treatment successes should be cause for the independent cancer community to rethink basic assumptions of molecular biology and cancer causation and prevention.

Statistics and statements from the National Cancer Institute show rising incidences of many cancers, including childhood brain cancer, breast cancer, skin cancer, lung cancer and colon cancer. And, when we do enjoy success, it is largely due to early detection and prevention efforts, which have been far more instrumental in fighting cancer than the harsh treatments that Big Pharma and the cancer establishment continue to advocate. In fact, if it were not for prevention and early diagnosis, treatments would be overwhelmed with greater failures.

But working without the insights and science that green molecular biologists now bring to the arena of cancer treatment and prevention is like trying to walk on one leg. Green is gentle, and in this case, subtle, yet it can work to amplify the benefits derived from the drugs of Big Pharma when, and if, the patient decides to integrate the two types of medicine: *allopathy* (conventional, Western medicine) and naturopathy (natural or holistic medicine).

A NEW VIEW

Beside the fact Dr. Mirko Beljanski was one of the very first to show the various roles of RNA in the cell (tumor-infectious RNA in plants, excreted RNA in showdomycin-resistant bacteria, transformant RNA in the bacteria, primer RNA boosting the immune system…) he also discovered that bacteria, eggs and fungus had a reverse transcriptase. At that time, only viruses were supposed to have such a fundamental enzyme, capable of overcoming the messages of DNA in cells.

Taking a completely original approach to carcinogenesis, he discovered a difference in DNA condensation of cancer cells, due, as he demonstrated, to the cumulative effect of carcinogens. He showed that many molecules in our environment behave as carcinogen-like molecules in this respect. In doing so, he was the first environmental researcher to activate the alarm bell with reference to pollution.

He devised a screening test for the dangerous molecules in the hope of finding a way to counteract them. Using this test (Oncotest), he found two plant extracts able to oppose DNA decondensation (destabilization of the secondary structure) and in so doing carcinogenesis. In fact, as it was largely confirmed later on, these two plant extracts prevent cancer cell multiplication, both *in vitro* and *in vivo*, without any effect on healthy cell multiplication. One of the two plant extracts also exhibited a powerful anti-viral activity.[19, 20]

All of these studies conducted by Beljanski led him to devise a new concept of carcinogenesis, a theoretical and practical approach that we have described in these pages.

Beljanski's findings in this vast area led him to new concepts of RNA's role, how various pathologies are initiated, but above all the importance of SELECTIVITY in biological activities.

In addition to the two plant extracts, he developed RNA fragments in order to enhance in a physiological manner, the *in vivo* production of white blood cells and platelets in people with immunosuppression. These RNA fragments act also selectively and exclusively on healthy cells.

He worked in a purely scientific manner on the fundamental cell mechanism.

A CLOSER LOOK

Beljanski believed DNA might help unlock the mystery of cancer. He peered into the very essence of life to study its intricacies. As we now know, the DNA molecule consists of two strands joined in a double helix: they draw apart from each other when the DNA must be copied as an identical DNA for the replication that is required prior to cell division, or transcribed as a messenger RNA for the synthesis of the proteins that are encoded in the genome.

The opening and the closing of the chain in relation to gene replication or expression are strictly regulated in the normal cell by distances between gaps of the bases in the helixes and other kinds of structural integrity.

Why then is the cancerous cell, as it undergoes rapid and anarchic division, able to synthesize molecules that normally it would not produce, thus escaping from strict cell regulation? Beljanski and his colleagues demonstrated how the DNA in cancerous cells is always "destabilized," that is, in many regions the two strands are spread apart from one another when they shouldn't be, leaving them susceptible to abnormal divisions and abnormal syntheses. This destabilized DNA is the very first stage of cancer and often appears before the occurrence of mutations. The destabilized DNA is left vulnerable to anything that is apt to increase its instability or "deregulated" activity. Thus, the precancerous or cancerous cell is extremely sensitive to carcinogens, which, as shown by Beljanski, also increase DNA instability.

But if there are substances which are capable of cumulatively triggering and maintaining destabilized DNA, might not there be others that would have the opposite effect? The research undertaken by Beljanski did in fact lead to the discovery of several molecules whose properties enabled them to intercalate onto the abnormally opened DNA chains, thus preventing the cancerous cells' survival. Such products work selectively: they do not act on healthy cells' DNA, leaving them free to pursue the course of their own division and synthesis.

In later phases of this research, Beljanski and his colleagues undertook to find the means of maintaining the right cell equilibrium, in terms of the enzymes that regulate DNA replication as well as the gene expression that it carries.

During the course of this research, they identified and developed several original efficacious and nontoxic plant-derived substances whose design is based on the physiological processes that occur normally in a healthy organism.

If Beljanski's name and work is indeed enjoying a renaissance among the leading experts now in the field of integrative medicine in America, it is because his work is great and solid and supplies real hope. This adaptation of his purely scientific and practical findings in America, where his work is being clinically and scientifically validated at major research institutions, is positively impacting our view on environmental toxicity and its consequences, as well as suggesting a way to shield ourselves at the DNA level.

Beljanski's research into the structural nature of DNA appears to be on the verge of profoundly changing the entire environmental carcinogenesis paradigm. His innovative approaches play a growing role in the complementary field of cancer treatment. He was the first to show that it is possible to selectively prevent precancer and cancer cells from developing without any incidence of toxicity to healthy cells.

Powerful green forces throughout the globe in science and medicine are causing science to re-examine the tenets Beljanski put forward—notably Donald Malins, Ph.D., whose work into the structure of DNA has revealed that DNA is indeed destabilized in cancer cells. And in 1989 in the journal *Nature* (December 7;342:624) the Nobel Prize winner Howard M. Temin, of the McArdle Laboratory, acknowledged Beljanski's own four earlier studies that led to the discovery of reverse transcriptase in prokaryotes, which is a very important result since it may also change the message carried by the DNA. Indeed, Mirko was first with this very relevant finding (since bacteria are considered to closely mirror a simplified version of human genetics), and the Temin retrocitation included his four seminal studies:

- Beljanski, M. *C. r. hebd. Séanc. Acad. Sci.*, Paris D274, 2801–2804 (1972).
- Beljanski, M. *C. r. hebd. Séanc. Acad. Sci.*, Paris D276, 1625–1628 (1973).
- Beljanski, M. & Beljanski, M. *Biochem. Genet.* 17, 163–180 (1974).
- Beljanski, M., Bourgarel, P. & Beljanski, M.S. *C. r. hebd. Séanc. Acad. Sci.*, Paris D286. 1825–1828 (1978).

His work has already become well-known in New York scientific circles. Research from the Columbia University Center for Holistic Urology and publications in peer-reviewed journals demonstrate promising results in clinical trials and other studies. A clinical trial at the Cancer Treatment Centers of America promises to revolutionize certain aspects of conventional cancer chemotherapy and radiation treatments, helping to make these widely accepted therapies more effective at prolonging life and fighting the disease. So it appears with this kind of biological and environmental approach, Beljanski's work is being fueled by the green movement within medicine and science, which is thankfully opening up the establishment to the possibilities that complementary medicine holds for all of us.

We are not proposing the superiority of naturopathy to allopathy, or conventional medicine, rather we contend that an integrative approach will ensure the best possible health outcome.

The first modern green scientist, Beljanski, through science and practical application, created real hope in the field of cancer prevention and treatment, and in other areas of environment and health. He was the first of the green molecular biologists to envision the rejoining of plants with modern allopathic medicine, not because he favored one over the other, but because he understood both could have positive influences on our health. No doubt, his balanced approach was rooted in his experience gleaned from the world of French socialized medicine, which provided treatment free of charge, but limited it to a few prescribed procedures, often with toxic side effects.

Beljanski brings hope through nature and science. There have been positive signs that we are surviving more types of cancers—but these victories stem mainly from early diagnosis and prevention. In some cases, doctors are embracing alternative medicine, as Beljanski understood it, not as the cure but as a more whole approach to the problem, as support for the healthy functions of the body when under stress. In this complementary approach, one speaks of shared benefits that enable the organism to live healthier and longer. He found unique and interesting plants from the rainforest and the African continent. He developed a noncellular assay for the detection of a substance's carcinogenic or preventive potential. He understood that there were assaults to the structure of DNA before mutations occurred, and that this was where the cell became sensitized to carcinogens and mutagens. His screening test could protect people from many pollutants if it were used to complement other critical cancer-screening tools like the Ames Test and experimental animal studies, cell cultures, and other test tube examinations.

Thus, we come to the work of a man who peered into the very secrets of life and brought to us another important scientific pathway that today is spawning an entirely new way of looking at health and the prevention and treatment of cancer and other degenerative diseases. Now we have a chance to re-examine cancer and its causes and prevention and perhaps reduce the toll it has taken on our population.

Here is the proposition: Science is walking on a well-trodden path devoting almost exclusive attention to genetic mutations in the information code, but another path, leading off the main one, passes through a different area with new discoveries to be made. This is the fundamental question that we pose: What if Beljanski were right all along? Don't we need to know to save our own lives?

Scientific Publications of Mirko Beljanski

1 A propos du microdosage du ribose dans les acides nucléiques et leurs dérivés:
   a) M. Beljanski, M. Macheboeuf, *C.R. Soc. Biol.* 1949, CXLIII, pp.174-175.
   b) M. Beljanski, *Ann. Inst. Pasteur*, 1949, 76, pp. 451-455.
2 F. Gros, M. Beljanski, M. Macheboeuf, F. Grumbach, "Comparaison biochimique d'une souche bactérienne sensible à la streptomycine avec une souche résistance de même espèce," *C.R. Acad. Sci.*, 1950, 230, pp. 875-877.
3 F. Gros, M. Beljanski, M. Macheboeuf, "Mode d'action de la pénicilline chez Staphylococcus aureus. Inhibition d'un système enzymatique extrait des bactéries," *C.R. Acad. Sci.*, 1950, 231, pp. 184-186.
4 F. Gros, M. Beljanski, M. Macheboeuf, "Action de la pénicilline sur le métabolisme de l'acide ribonucléique chez *Staphylococcus aureus*," *Bull. Soc. Chim. Biol.*, 1951, 33, pp.1696-1717.
5 F. Gros, M. Beljanski, M. Macheboeuf, F. Grumbach, F. Boyer, "Activité biologique des combinaisons streptomycine-acides gras," *C.R. Acad., Sci.*, 1951, 232, pp.764-766.
6 M. Beljanski, "Etude de souches bactériennes résistantes à des antibiotiques. Comparaison avec des souches sensibles de mêmes espèces," *Ann. Biol.*, 1951, 27, pp. 775-780.
7 M. Beljanski, "Etude des souches bactériennes résistantes à des antibiotiques. Comparaison avec des souches sensibles de mêmes espèces," Thèse de Doctorat ès Sciences d'Etat, Université Paris-la Sorbonne, 1951, Paris, Librairie Arnette, 1952.

8 M. Beljanski, "Action de la cocarboxylase sur le métabolisme des acides nucléiques chez *Staphylococcus aureus* sensible et résistant à la streptomycine," 2ème Congrès Intern. de Biochimie, Paris, 1952. *Résumé des communications,* 99.

9 M. Beljanski, "Comparaison de souches bactériennes résistantes à des antibiotiques avec des souches sensibles de même espèce - I : Cas de la streptomycine," *Ann. Inst. Pasteur*, 1952, 83, pp. 80-101.

10 M. Beljanski, "Comparaison de souches bactériennes résistantes à des antibiotiques avec des souches sensibles de même espèce - II : Cas de la pénicilline," *Ann. Inst. Pasteur*, 1953, 84, pp. 402-408.

11 M. Beljanski, "Comparaison de souches bactériennes résistantes à des antibiotiques avec des souches sensibles de même espèce - III : Cas du sulfamide - IV : Cas de l'azoture de sodium," *Ann. Inst. Pasteur,* 1953, 84, pp. 756-764.

12 M. Beljanski, "Comparaison de souches bactériennes résistantes à la streptomycine avec des souches sensibles de même espèce," *C.R. Acad. Sci.*, 1953, 236, pp. 1102-1104.

13 M. Beljanski, F. Grumbach, "Etude biochimique d'une souche de Mycobacterium tuberculosis streptomycino-sensible et d'une souche streptomycino-résistance dérivée de la souche sensible," *C.R. Acad., Sci.*, 1953, 236, pp. 2111-2113.

14 M. Beljanski, "Etude des acides nucléiques de souches bactériennes résistantes à la streptomycine et souches de mêmes espèces mais sensibles à l'antibiotique," *Ann. Inst. Pasteur*, 1953, 85, pp. 463-469.

15 M. Beljanski, J.Guelfi, "Etude à l'aide du 32P de l'accumulation des acides nucléiques chez *Staphylococcus aureus* et *Salmonella enteritidis* résistants et sensibles à la streptomycine," *Ann. Inst. Pasteur*, 1954, 86, pp. 115-117.

16 M. Beljanski, "L'absence de cytochromes et de certains systèmes enzymatiques dans un nouveau mutant d'*Escherichia coli* streptomycino-résistant. Comparaison avec la souche sensible dont il dérive," *C.R. Acad., Sci.*, 1954, 238, pp. 852-854.

17 M. Beljanski, "L'action de la ribonucléase et de la désoxyribonucléase sur l'incorporation de glycocolle radioactif dans les protéines de lysats de *Micrococcus lysodeikticus*," *Biochim. Biophys. Acta.* 15, 99. 425-431.

18 M. Beljanski, "Isolement de mutants d'*Escherichia coli* streptomycino-résistants dépourvus d'enzymes respiratoires. Action de l'hémine sur la formation de ces enzymes chez le mutant H-7," *C.R. Acad., Sci.*, 1955, 240, pp. 374-376.

19 M. Beljanski, "Formation d'enzymes respiratoires chez un mutant d'*Escherichia coli* streptomycino-résistant ne manifestant pas d'activité respiratoire," 3ème Congrès Intern. Biochim., Bruxelles, 1955, p. 98 - Résumés des communications.

20 R. Latarjet, M. Beljanski, "Photorestoration in porphyrin-less mutants of *Escherichia coli*," *Microbial Genetic Bulletin*, E. Witkin, 1955 - Résumés.

21 M. Beljanski, "Reconstitution *in vitro* de la catalase," *C.R. Acad., Sci.*, 1955, 241, pp. 1353-1355.

22 R. Latarjet, M. Beljanski, "Photorestauration de bactéries dépourvues de porphyrines," *Ann. Inst. Pasteur*, 1956, 90, pp. 127-132.

23 M. Beljanski, M. S. Beljanski, "Sur la formation d'enzymes respiratoires chez un mutant d'*Escherichia coli* streptomycino-résistant et auxotrophe pour l'hémine," *Ann. Inst. Pasteur*, 1957, 92, pp. 396-412.

24 M. Beljanski, S. Ochoa, "Protein bio-synthesis by a cell-free bacterial system," *Proc. Nat. Acad. Sci. Biochemistry*, 1958, 44, pp. 494-500.

25 M. Beljanski, M. S. Beljanski, VII-ème Congrès Intern. de Microbiol. Stockholm, 1958, Symposium, II. Discussions.

26 M. Beljanski, S. Ochoa, "Protein bio-synthesis by a cell-free bacterial system," *IV-ème Congrès Intern. Biochim. Vienne*, 1958, p. 49 - Résumés des communications.

27 M. Beljanski, S. Ochoa, "Protein bio-synthesis by a cell-free bacterial system. II-Further studies on the amino acid incorporation enzyme," *Proc. Nat. Acad. Sci.*, 1958, 44, pp. 1157-1161.

28 M. Beljanski, "Identification de quatre kinases spécifiques des diphosphonucléosides dans une préparation enzymatique d'origine bactérienne," *C.R. Acad. Sci.*, 1959, 248, pp. 1146-1448.

29 M. Beljanski, "Synthèse de peptides par un système enzymatique en présence de nucléoside - triphosphates," *C.R. Acad. Sci.*, 1960, 250, pp. 624-626.

30 M. Beljanski, "Protein biosynthesis by a cell-free bacterial system. III-Determination of new peptide bonds; requirements for the amino acid incorporation enzyme in protein biosynthesis," *Biochim. Biophys. Acta.*, 1960, 41, pp. 104-110.

31 M. Beljanski, "Protein biosynthesis by a cell-free bacterial system. IV-Exchange of diphosphonucleosides with homologous triphosphonucleosides by the amino acid incorporation enzyme," *Biochim. Biophys. Acta.*, 1960, 41, pp. 111-115.

32 M. Beljanski, "Ribonucleoside-5'-triphosphate dependent synthesis of peptides by the purified amino acid incorporation enzyme," *Progress in Biophysics and Biophysical Chemistry*, Pergamon Press, 1961, 11, p. 238.

33 M. Beljanski, "Ribonucléoside-triphosphates et synthèses de peptides spécifiques par des enzymes purifiés," *Bull. Soc. Chim. Biol.*, 1961,43, pp. 1018-1030.

34 M. Beljanski, "Ribonucléoside-triphosphates et synthèse enzymatique de liaisons peptidiques," Symposium sur les Acides Ribonucléiques et les Polyphosphates," C.N.R.S., 1961, pp. 474-475.

35 M. Beljanski, M. S. Beljanski, "Synthèses de peptides spécifiques par un système enzymatique purifié d'*Alcaligenes faecalis*," Vème Congrès Intern. Biochim. Moscou, 1961, p. 24.

36 M. Beljanski, Discussions, Symposium sur la Biosynthèse des Protéines. Vème Congrès Intern. Biochim. Moscou, 1961.

37 J.P. Zalta, M. Beljanski, "Synthèse de peptides par des fractions subcellulaires préparées à partir du foie de rat," *C.R. Acad. Sci.* 1961, 253, pp. 567-569.

38 M. Beljanski, M. S. Beljanski, T. Loviny, "Rôle des polypeptide-synthétases dans la formation de peptides spécifiques en présence de ribonucléoside-triphosphates," *Biochim. Biophys. Acta.*, 1962, 56, pp. 559-570.

39 M. Beljanski, "Participation of an RNA fraction in peptide synthesis in the presence of a purified enzyme system from *Alcaligenes faecalis*," *Biochim. Biophys. Res. Comm.*, 1962, 8, pp. 15-19.

40 M. Beljanski, M.S. Beljanski, "Acide aminé - acide ribonucléique, intermédiaire dans la synthèse des liasons peptidiques," VI- *Biochim. Biophys. Acta.*, 1963, 72, pp. 585-597.

41 M. Beljanski, "ARN-messager: intermédiaire direct dans la synthèse des liaisons peptidiques," Colloque International du C.N.R.S., Marseille, 1963, pp. 39-44. (Mécanismes de régulation des activités cellulaires chez les micro-organismes).

42 M. Beljanski, C. Fisher, M.S. Beljanski, "Le RNA messager, accepteur spécifique des L-acides aminés en présence d'enzymes bactériennes," *C.R. Acad. Sci.*, 1963,257, pp. 547-549.

43 M. Beljanski, C. Fisher, "Les ARN messagers gouvernant la synthèse *in vitro* des chaînes peptidiques en présence de polypeptides synthétases," *Pathologie-Biologie*, 1965,13, pp. 198-203.

44 M. Beljanski, "Messenger RNA dependent Synthesis of peptides by purified bacterial enzymes." *Bioch-Zeits*, 1965, 342, pp. 392-399.

45 M. Beljanski, "L'ARN isolé du virus de la mosaïque jaune du Navet, accepteur des l-acides aminés en présence d'enzymes bactériennes," *Bull. Soc. Chim. Biol.* 1965, 47, pp. 1645-1652.

46 M. Beljanski, N. Vapaille, "Rôle des triterpènes dans l'attachement des l-acides aminés par des ARN matriciels," *Eur. J. of Clin. Biol. Res.*, 1971, pp. 897-908.

47 M. Beljanski, P. Bourgarel, "Isolement de di- et trinucléotides, sites spécifiques d'attachement d'arginine et de valine dans des ARN d' origines différentes," *C.R. Acad. Sci.*, 1967, 264, pp. 1760-1763 (série D).

48 M. Beljanski, C. Fischer-Ferraro, "Nouvelle méthode de purification des polypeptides synthétases," *C.R. Acad. Sci.*, 1967, 264, pp. 411-414 (série D).

49 M. Beljanski, C. Fischer-Ferraro, P. Bourgarel, "Identification des sites d'attachement spécifiques d'arginine et de valine dans des ARN d' origines différentes," VIII- European *J. Biochem.*, 1968, 4, pp. 184-189.

50 C. Fischer-Ferraro, M. Beljanski, "Nouvelle méthode de purification des polypeptides synthétases," VII- European *J. Biochem.*, 1968, 4, pp. 118-125.

51 M. Beljanski, P. Bourgarel, "Isolement et caractérisation d'un RNA matriciel d'*Alcaligenes faecalis*," *C.R. Acad. Sci.*, 1968, 266, pp. 845-847.

52 M. Beljanski, M.S. Beljanski, "Synthèse chez *Escherichia coli* des ARN dont la structure primaire diffère de celle de l'ADN," *C.R. Acad. Sci.*, 1968, 267, pp. 1058-1060 (série D).

53 M. Beljanski, M.S. Beljanski, P. Bourgarel, J. Chassagne, "Synthèse chez les bactéries d'ARN nouveaux n'étant pas la copie de l'ADN," *C.R. Acad. Sci.*, 1969, 269, pp. 240-243 (série D).

54 M. Beljanski, P. Bourgarel, M.S. Beljanski, "Showdomycine et biosynthèse d'ARN non complémentaire de l'ADN," - I -. *Ann. Inst. Pasteur*, 1970, 118, pp. 253-276.

55 M. Beljanski, P. Bourgarel, M.S. Beljanski, "Drastic alteration of ribosomal RNA and ribosomal proteins in showdomycin-resistant *Escherichia coli*," *Proc. Nat. Aca. Sci.* (USA), 1971,68, pp. 491-495.

56 M. Plawecki, M. Beljanski, "Transcription par la polynucléotide phosphorylase de l'ARN associé à l'ADN d'*Escherichia coli*," *C.R. Acad. Sci.*, 1971, 273, pp. 827-830 (série D).

57 M. Beljanski, M.S. Beljanski, P. Bourgarel, "ARN transformants porteurs de caractères héréditaires chez *Escherichia coli* showdomycino-résistant," *C.R. Acad. Sci.*, 1971, 272, pp. 2107-2110 (série D).

58 M. Beljanski, M.S. Beljanski, P. Bourgarel, "Episome à ARN porté par l'ADN d'*Escherichia coli* sauvage et showdomycino-résistant," *C.R. Acad. Sci.*, 1971, 272, pp. 2736-3739 (série D).

59 M. Beljanski, M.S. Beljanski, P. Manigault, P. Bourgarel, "Transformation of *Agrobacterium tumefaciens* into a non-oncogenic species by an *Escheria coli* RNA," *Proc. Nat. Aca. Sci.* (USA), 1972, 69, pp. 191-195.

60 M. Beljanski, "Synthèse *in vitro* de l'ADN sur une matrice d'ARN par une transcriptase d'*Escherichia coli*," *C.R. Acad. Sci.*, 1972, 274, pp.2801-2804 (série D).

61 M. Beljanski, C. Bonissol, P. Kona, "Transformation des cellules K.B. induites par la showdomycine," *C.R. Acad. Sci.*, 1972,274, pp. 3116-3119 (série D).

62 M. Beljanski, P. Manigault, "Genetic transformation of bacteria by RNA and loss of oncogenic power properties of *Agrobacterium tumefaciens*. Transforming RNA as template for DNA synthesis," *Sixth Miles International Symposium on Molecular Biology*. Ed. F. Beers and R.C. Tilghman. The John Hopkins University Press, Baltimore, 1972, pp. 81-97.

63 M. Beljanski, "Séparation de la transcriptase inverse de l'ADN polymérase ADN dépendante. Analyse de l'ADN synthétisé sur le modèle de l'ARN transformant," *C.R. Acad. Sci.*, 1973, 276, pp. 1625-1628 (série D).

64 M. Beljanski, M. Plawecki, "Transforming RNA as a template directing RNA and DNA synthesis in bacteria," In Niu and Segal (eds), *The Role of RNA in Reproduction and Development*. North Holland Publ.Co., 1973, pp. 203-224.

65 M. Plawecki, M. Beljanski, "Synthèse *in vitro* d'un ARN utilisé comme amorceur pour la réplication de l'ADN," *C.R. Acad. Sci.*, 1974, 278, pp. 1413-1416 (série D).

66 M. Beljanski, Y. Aaron-Da-Cunha, M.S. Beljanski, P. Manigault, P. Bourgarel, "Isolation of the tumor-inducing RNA from Oncogenic and Nononcogenic *Agrobacterium tumefaciens*," *Proc. Nat. Acad. Sci.* (USA), 1974,71, pp. 1585-1589.

67 M. Beljanski, M.S. Beljanski, "RNA-bound Reverse Transcriptase in *Escherichia coli* and *in vitro* synthesis of a complementary DNA," *Biochemical genetics*, 1974, 12, pp. 163-180.

68 M. Beljanski, P. Manigault, M.S. Beljanski, Y. Aaron-Da-Cunha, "Genetic transformation of *Agrobacterium tumefaciens* by RNA and nature of the tumor inducing principle," First Intern. Congress of the *Intern. Assoc. of Microbiol. Soc.* Tokyo I.A.M.S., 1974,1, pp.132-141.

69 M. Beljanski, M. S. Beljanski, M. Plawecki, P. Manigault, "ARN-fragments, amorceurs nécessaires à la réplication *in vitro* des ADN," *C.R. Acad. Sci.,* 1975,280, pp. 363-366 (série D).

70 M. Beljanski, L. Chaumont, C. Bonissol, M. S. Beljanski, "ARN-fragments inhibiteurs *in vivo* de la multiplication des virus du fibrome de Shope et de la vaccine," *C.R. Acad. Sci.,* 1975, 280, pp. 783-786 (série D).

71 M. Beljanski, "ARN-amorceurs riches en nucléotides G et A indispensables à la réplication *in vitro* de l'ADN des phages YX174 et lambda," *C.R. Acad. Sci.,* 1975, 280, pp. 783-786 (série D).

72 L. Le Goff, Y. Aaron-Da-Cunha, M. Beljanski, "RNA fraction from several nononcogenic strains of *Agrobacterium tumefaciens* as tumor inducing agent in *Datura stramonium*," XIIth Intern. Bot. Congress. Résumés. Leningrad, 1975.

73 M. Beljanski, Y. Aaron-Da-Cunha, "RNA fraction from others sources than *Agrobacterium tumefaciens* as tumor inducing agent in *Datura stramonium*," Workshop Third Intern. Congress of Virology, Madrid, 1975, p. 15.

74 L. Le Goff Y. Aaron-Da-Cunha, M. Beljanski, "Un ARN extrait d'*Agrobacterium tumefaciens* souches oncogènes et non oncogènes, éléments indispensables à l'induction des tumeurs chez *Datura stramonium*," *Canadian J. of Microbiology*, 1976, 22, pp. 694-701.

75 M. Beljanski, Y. Aaron-Da-Cunha, "Particular small size RNA and RNA fragments from different origins as tumor inducing agents in in Datura stramoium," *Molec. Biol. Reports*, 1976, 2, pp. 497-506.

76 S.K. Dutta, M. Beljanski, P. Bourgarel, "Endogenous RNA-bound RNA dependent DNA polymerase activity in *Neurospora crassa*," *Exp. Mycology*, 1977, 1, pp. 173-182.

77 L. Le Goff, Y. Aaron-Da-Cunha, M. Beljanski, "Polyribonucleotides, agents inducteurs et inhibiteurs des tissus tumoraux," Conf. Intern. Montpellier (1978) - Résumés.

78 M. Beljanski, P. Bourgarel, M.S. Beljanski, "Découpage des ARN ribo-somiques d'*Escherichia coli* par la ribonucléase U2 et transcription *in vitro* des ARN-fragments en ADN complémentaires," *C.R. Acad. Sci.*, 1978, 286, pp. 1825-1828 (série D).

79 M. Beljanski, M. Plawecki, P. Bourgarel, M. S. Beljanski, "Nouvelles sub-stances (R.L.B.) actives dans la leucopoïese et la formation des plaquettes," *Bull. Acad. Nat. Med.*, 1978, 162, Volume n°6, pp. 475-781.

80 M. Stroun, Ph. Anker, M. Beljanski, J. Henri, Ch. Lederrey, M. Ojha, P. Maurice, "Presence of RNA in the nucleo-protein complex spontaneously released by human lymphocytes and frog auricles," *Cancer Res.*, 1978, 38, pp. 3546-3551.

81 M. Beljanski, L. Le Goff, Y. Aaron-Da-Cunha, "Special short dual-action RNA fragments can both induce and inhibit crown-gall tumors," Proc. 4th Conf. Plant Path. Bacteria Angers, 1978, pp. 207-220.

82 M. Beljanski, L. Le Goff, "Stimulation de l'induction - ou inhibition du développement - des tumeurs de crown-gall par des ARN-fragments U2. Interférence de l'auxine," *C.R. Acad. Sci.*, 1979, 288, pp. 147-150 (série D).

83 M. Beljanski, M. Plawecki, "Particular RNA fragments as promoters of leuco-cytes and platelet formations in rabbits," *Exp. Cell Biol.*, 1979, 47, pp. 218-225.

84 M. Beljanski, "Oncotest: a DNA assay system for the screening of carcino-genic substances," IRCS Medical Science, 1979, 47, pp. 218-225.

85 L. Le Goff, M. Beljanski, "Cancer/anti-cancer dual action drugs in crown-gall tumors," *IRCS Medical Science*, 1979,7, p. 476.

86 M. Beljanski, "Oligoribo-nucleotides, promoters of leucocyte and platelet genesis in animals depleted by anticancer drugs," NCI-EORTC Symposium on nature, prevention and treatment of clinical toxicity of anticancer agents. Institut Bordet, Bruxelles, 1980.

87 M. Beljanski, M. Plawecki, P. Bourgarel, M.S. Beljanski, "Short chain RNA fragments as promoters of leucocyte and platelet genesis in animals depleted by anti-cancer drugs," *In the Role of RNA in Development and Reproduction.* Sec. Int. Symposium, April 25-30, 1980, pp. 79-113. Science Press Beijing. M.C. Niu and H.H. Chuang Eds Van Nostrand Reinhold Company.

88 M. Beljanski, P. Bourgarel, M.S. Beljanski, "Correlation between *in vitro* DNA synthesis, DNA strand separation and *in vivo* multiplication of cancer cells," *Expl. Cell. Biol.*, 49,1981, pp.220-231.

89 M. Plawecki, M. Beljanski, "Comparative study of *Escherichia coli* endotoxin, hydrocortisone and Beljanski Leucocyte Restorers activity in cyclophosphamide-treated rabbits," *Proc. of the Soc. for Exp. Biol. and Med.*, 168, 1981, pp.408-413.

90 M. Beljanski, L. Le Goff, M.S. Beljanski, "Differential susceptibility of cancer and normal DNA templates allows the detection of carcinogens and anticancer drugs," Third NCI-EORTS Symp. on new drugs in Cancer Therapy, Institut Bordet, Bruxelles, 1981.

91 L. Le Goff, M. Beljanski, "Crown-gall tumor stimulation or inhibition: correlation with DNA strand separation," *Proc. Fifth Conf. Plant Path. Bact. Cali*, 1981, p. 295-307.

92 M. Beljanski, M.S. Beljanski, "Selective inhibition of *in vitro* synthesis of cancer DNA by alkaloids of b-carboline class," *Expl. Cell. Biol.*, 50, 1982, pp.79-87.

93 L. Le Goff, M. Beljanski, "Agonist and/or antagonists effects of plant hormones and an anticancer alkaloid on plant structure and activity," *IRCS Med. Sci.*, 10, 1982, pp. 689-690.

94 M. Beljanski, L. Le Goff, A. Faivre-Amiot, "Preventive and curative anticancer drug. Application to Crown-gall tumors," *Acta Horticulturae*, n°125, 1982, pp. 239-248.

95 M. Beljanski, "Oncotest: dépistage des potentiels cancérogènes et spécifiquement cancéreux. Conceptions et perspectives nouvelles en cancérologie," *Environnement et nouvelle médecine.* n°2, 1982, pp.18-23.

96 M. Beljanski, L. Le Goff, M. S. Beljanski, "*In vitro* Screening of Carcinogens using DNA of the His-Mutant of *Salmonella typhimurium*," *Expl. Cell. Biol.*, 50, 1982, pp. 271-280.

97 M. Beljanski, L. Le Goff, "Tumor promoter (TPA), DNA chain opening and unscheduled DNA synthesis," *IRCS Med. Sci.*, 11, 1983, pp. 363-364.

98 M. Beljanski, M. Plawecki, P. Bourgarel, M.S. Beljanski, "Leucocyte recovery whith short-chain RNA fragments in cyclophosphamide-treated rabbits," *Cancer Treatment Reports,* 67, 1983, pp. 611-619.

99 M. Beljanski, "The Regulation of DNA Replication and Transcription. The Role of Trigger Molecules in Normal and Malignant Gene Expression," *Experimental Biology and Medicine*, vol. 8, Karger (1983), pp. 1-190.

100 M. Beljanski, M.S. Beljanski, "Three alkaloids as selective destroyers of the proliferative capacity of cancer cells," *IRCS Med. Sci.*, 12, 1984, pp. 587-588.

101 L. Le Goff, J. Roussaux, Y. Aaron-Da-Cunha, M. Beljanski, "Growth inhibition of crown-gall tissues in relation to the structure and activity of DNA," *Physiol. Plant.*, 64, 1985, pp 177-184.

102 L. Le Goff, M. Beljanski, "The *in vitro* effects of opines and other compounds on DNAs originating from bacteria and from healthy and tumorous plant tissues," *Expl. Cell. Biol.*, 53, 1985, pp. 335-350.

103 M. Beljanski, "Activation et inactivation des gènes: Incidence en cancérologie," *Aspect de la recherche*. Université Paris-Sud, 1985, pp. 56-62.

104 M. Beljanski, M.S. Beljanski, "Three alkaloids as selective destroyers of cancer cells in mice. Synergy with classic anticancer drugs," *Oncology*, 43, 1986, pp 198-203.

105 M. Beljanski, L. Le Goff, "Analysis of small RNA species: phylogenetic trends," *In DNA Systematics, vol.I: Evolution*. Ed. S.K. Dutta CRC Press, Inc. Florida (1986), pp.81-105.

106 M. Beljanski, T. Nawrocki, L. Le Goff, "Possible role of markers synthesized during cancer evolution: I- Markers in mamalian tissues," *IRCS Med. Sci.* 14, 1986, pp. 809-810.

107 L. Le Goff, M. Beljanski, "Possible role of markers synthesized during cancer evolution: II- Markers in crown-gall tissues," *IRCS Med. Sci.* 14, 1986, pp. 811-812.

108 M. Beljanski, L. Le Goff, M.S. Beljanski, "Régulation des gènes, cancer et prévention," *Médecines nouvelles*, 15, 1986, pp. 57-86.

109 M. Beljanski, "Terminal deoxynucleotidyl transferase and ribonuclease activities in purified hepatitis-B antigen," *Med. Sci. Res.*, 15, 1987, pp. 529-530.

110 M. Beljanski, S.K. Dutta, "Differential synthesis and replication of DNA in the *Neurospora crassa* slime mutant versus normal cells: Role of carcinogens," *Oncology*, 44, 1987, pp. 327-330.

111 S.K. Dutta, M. Beljanski, "Particular RNA primer from growth medium differentially stimulates *in vitro* DNA synthesis and *in vivo* cell growth of *Neurospora crassa* and its slime mutant," *Current Genetics*, 12, 1987, pp. 283-289.

112 M. Beljanski, L.C. Niu, M.S. Beljanski, S. Yan, M.C. NIU, "Iron stimulated RNA-dependent DNA polymerase Activity from goldfish eggs," *Cellular and Molecular Biology*, 34, 1988, pp. 17-25.

113 L. Le Goff, M. Wicker, M. Beljanski, "Reversible biophysical changes of DNAs from *in vitro* culturel non-tumour cells," *Med. Sci. Res.*, 16, 1988, pp. 359-360.

114 M. Stroun, P. Anker, P. Maurice, J. Lyautey, C. Lederrey, M. Beljanski, "Neoplastic Characteristics of the DNA Found in the Plasma of Cancer Patients," *Oncology*, 16, 1989, pp. 318-322.

115 M. Beljanski, M.S. Beljanski, M. Grandi "Resultati preliminari dell'impiego di tre alcaloidi nel carcinoma prostatico," *In Tumori, Instituo Nationale per le studio ed la cura dei tumori* (ed. Lambrosiana), Vol. 75, suppl. 4, 1989.

116 M. Beljanski, "Cancer therapy: A New Approach," *Deutsche Zeitschrift für Onkologie* 5, 22, 1990, pp. 145-152.

117 M. Beljanski, "Cancer et Sida. Nouvelles approches thérapeutiques," *5èmes Entretiens Internationaux de Monaco*, 21-24 novembre 1990 (Ed. du Rocher), pp. 25-34.

118 D. Donadio, R. Lorho, J.E. Causse, T. Nawrocki, M. Beljanski, "RNA fragments (RLB) and Tolerance of Cytostatic Treatments in Hematology: A Preliminary Study about Two Non-Hodgkin Malignant Lymphoma Cases," *Deutsche Zeitschrift für Onkologie*, 23, 2, 1991, pp. 33-35.

119 M. Beljanski, "Reverse Transcriptases in Bacteria: Small RNAs as Genetic Vectors and Biological Modulators," *Brazil. J. Genetics*, 14, 4, 1991, pp. 873-896.

120 M. Beljanski, "Radioprotection of Irradiated Mice - Mechanisms and Synergistic Action of WR-2721 and R.L.B.," *Deutsche Zeitschrift für Onkologie*, 23, 6, 1991, pp. 155-159.

121 M. Beljanski, "Overview: BLRs as Inducers of *in vivo* Leucocyte and Platelet Genesis," *Deutsche Zeitschrift für Onkologie*, 24, 2, 1992, pp. 45-45.

122 M. Beljanski, "A New Approach to Cancer Therapy," *Proceedings of the international seminar: Traditional Medicine: A Challenge of the 21st Century*, 7-9 Nov. 1992, Calcutta (Ed. in chief Biswapati Mukherjee).

123 M. Beljanski, S. Crochet, M.S. Beljanski, "PB100: A Potent and Selective Inhibitor of Human BCNU Resistant Glioblastoma Cell Multiplication," *Anticancer Research*, vol. 13, n°6A, Nov. Dec. 1993, pp. 2301-2308.

124 M. Beljanski, S. Crochet, "Differential effects of ferritin, calcium, zinc and gallic acid on *in vitro* proliferation of human glioblastoma cells and normal astrocytes," *J. Lab. Clin. Med.* 123:547-555, 1994.

125 M. Beljanski, S. Crochet, "The selective anticancer agent PB-100 inhibits interleukin-6 induced enhancement of glioblastoma cell proliferation *in vitro*," *International Journal of Oncology*, 5:873-879, 1994.

126 M. Beljanski, S. Crochet, "Selective inhibitor (PB-100) of human glioblastoma cell multiplication," *Journal of Neuro-Oncology*, Vol. 21, N°1, p. 62, 1994.

127 J.E. Causse, T. Nawrocki, M. Beljanski, "Human Skin Fibrosis Rnase Search for a Biological Inhibitor-Regulator," *Deutsche Zeitschrift für Onkologie*, 26, 5, 1994, pp. 137-139.

128 M. Beljanski, S. Crochet, "The anticancer agent PB100 concentrates in the nucleus and nucleoli of human glioblastoma cells but does not enter normal astrocytes," *International Journal of Oncology* 7:81-85, 1995.

129 M. Beljanski, "Novel selective nontoxic anticancer and antiviral agents," *International Journal of Oncology* Vol. 7. supplement, p. 983, October 1995.

130 M. Beljanski, S. Crochet, "The selective anticancer agents PB-100 and BG-8 are active against human melanoma cells, but do not affect non malignant fibroblasts," *International Journal of Oncology* 8:1143-1148, 1996.

131 M. Beljanski, S. Crochet, "Mitogenic effect of several interleukins, neurome-diators and hormones on human glioblastoma cells, and its inhibition by the selective anticancer agent PB-100," *Deutsche Zeitschrift für Onkologie*, 28, 1, 1996, pp. 14-2.

132 M. Beljanski, "De novo synthesis of DNA - like molecules by polyaudeotide phosphorylase *in vitro*," *J. Mol. Evol.* 1996, 42:493-499.

133 M. Beljanski, "The anticancer agent PB-100, selectively active on malignant cells, inhibits multiplication of sixteen malignant cell lines, even multidrug resistant," *Genetics and Molecular Biology*, 23, 1, 29-33 (2000).

Beljanski's Time Line

A. EARLY STUDIES

1947-1954
- Bi Biochemical studies comparing sensitive strains of bacteria and ones resistant to various antibiotics.
- Accumulation of ribonucleic acids at the time of the resistance (references 1 to 17).

1955-1957
- Studies of the loss of respiratory enzymes in certain bacteria resistant to antibiotics.
- Reconstruction of these enzymes by the catalase.
- Photo-restoration of the cellular lesions produced by the U.V. rays in two mutants, thanks to peroxidases (references 18 to 23).

1958-1968
- Attempting to understand the role of transfer RNA and the genetic code.
- How particular RNAs from viral sources intervene in peptide synthesis.
- Importance of RNAs in vital mechanisms (references 24 to 50).

B. MID-LIFE STUDIES

1972
- **Discovery of transformant RNA**, excreted by *E.coli* resistant to showdomycin.
- Study of the origin, synthesis and characteristics of this RNA.
- Loss of the oncogenic properties of *A. tumefaciens* once transformed by this RNA.
- First example in biology that RNA can cause a stable, hereditary genetic transformation.

• Transforming RNA as a template directing RNA and DNA synthesis in bacteria (references 52, 53, 54, 55, 56, 57, 58, 59, 62, 64, 65, 66, 68).

• **Discovery of Reverse-Transcriptase** in bacteria (references 60, 62, 63, 64, 67).
• Reverse-Transcriptase in *Neurospora crassa* (ref 76).
  In goldfish eggs: (ref 112).

• **Small RNAs** of different nature and origin play different roles in biology:
  – as inhibitors of viral tumors in rabbits (reference 70).
  – as tumor-inducing RNA in plants (references 66, 68, 72, 73, 74, 75, 77).
  – as inhibitors of plant tumors (references 78, 81, 82, 85).
  – as primers for DNA replication of two bacteriophages (reference 71).
  – synthesis *in vitro* of an RNA primer (reference 65).

• **RNA primers for DNA bone marrow replication.** New studies *in vitro* and *in vivo*.
• Production of white blood cells and platelets in immuno-depleted animals & humans (references 79, 80, 83, 86, 87, 89, 98, 105, 111, 118, 121), overview (reference 121).

• **Oncotest.** Destabilization of DNA in cancer tissues.
• Screening of carcinogens and carcinogen-like molecules (references 84, 95).
• Oncotest in plants (references 90, 91).
• Destabilization of the DNA. Correlation with DNA synthesis, DNA strand.
• Separation and cancer cell multiplication (references 88, 90, 91, 93, 97).
• Application of Oncotest to the His-Mutant of *Salmonella typhimurium* (Ames test) (reference 96).

• **Selective plant molecules:** *Rauwolfia vomitoria* and Pao pereira.
• Identification of active molecules. Characteristics (references 85, 92, 93, 94).
• Studies *in vitro* (references 88, 90, 92, 100, 123, 125, 126, 128, 130, 131, 133).
  − *in vivo* on plants (references 85, 91, 93, 94).
  − on mice grafted with many different lines of cancer cells (references 104). Mice are treated by different routes with anti-cancer drugs alone or in synergy with classical chemotherapies.
• Biochemical, toxicological studies.

• **Influence of the Environment** (references 93, 97, 99, 102, 106, 107, 108, 109, 112, 124).

C. LATE STUDIES

1990-2000   • Proposition of a new approach to cancer therapy (references 116, 117, 121, 122).

• **Radioprotection studies**
• Development of the *Ginkgo biloba* extract (references 120, 127).

• **De novo synthesis of DNA** (reference 132).

Resources

The Beljanski Foundation, Inc., a not-for-profit organization, was vested with the mission of furthering the research begun nearly fifty years ago by molecular biologist Mirko Beljanski, Ph.D., at the Pasteur Institute in Paris, France. The research started by Dr. Beljanski remains rich in potential discovery. The Foundation remains committed to supporting further study of scientific concepts and discoveries made by Dr. Beljanski.

To learn more about the Beljanski Foundation, visit www.beljanski.com.

TO LOCATE A CAM PHYSICIAN

To locate a doctor who uses the Beljanski plant extracts, visit the American College for Advancement in Medicine and use their physician referral service at

- www.acam.org.

The International College of Integrative Medicine:
- 122 Thurman St. Box 271, Bluffton, OH 45817
- www.icimed.com
- (419) 358-0273

Visit Michael Schachter, M.D., at the following:
- www.schachtercenter.com
- www.mbschachter.com

To contact the office, call (845) 368-4700, fax (845) 368-4727, or e-mail office@mbschachter.com.

Visit also www.canhelp.com for additional CAM information.

For information on Cancer Treatment Centers of America,
visit www.cancercenters.com or call (800) 268-0786.

References

1   Brachet, J. "Exposé: Souvenirs sur les origines de la biologie moléculaire." *Bull CI Sci Acad R Belg*, 1987;73:441-449.

2   See, for example, Goudot, A. "Aspect electronique de la formation de mutants par certains antibiotiques." *Cahiers de Physique*, 1967;201:191-199.

3   Beljanski, M. & Manigault, P. In: Beers, F. and Tilghman, R. C. (eds.), *Genetic Transformation of Bacteria by RNA and Loss of Oncogenic Power Properties of Agrobacterium tumefaciens. Transforming RNA as Template for DNA Synthesis.* Sixth Miles International Symposium on Molecular Biology. Baltimore: The John Hopkins University Press, 1972.

4   Beljanski, M. & Plawecki, M. In: Niu and Segal (eds.), *Transforming RNA as a Template Directing RNA and DNA Synthesis in Bacteria. The Role of RNA in Reproduction and Development.* Amsterdam: North Holland Publ. Co., 1973.

5   Beljanski, M., et al. "Isolation of the tumor-inducing RNA from oncogenic and nononcogenic *Agrobacterium tumefaciens*." *Proc Nat Acad Sci*, 1974:1585-1589.

6   Beljanski, M. "Synthèse *in vitro* de l'ADN sur une matrice d'ARN par une transcriptase d'*Escherichia coli*." *CR Acad Sci*, 1972;274:2801-2804.

7   Beljanski, M., et al. "Transformation des cellules K.B. induites par la showdomycine." *CR Acad Sci*, 1972;274:3116-3119.

8   Beljanski, M. & Manigault, P., Op cit.

9   Beljanski, M. "Séparation de la transcriptase inverse de l'ADN polymérase ADN dépendante. Analyse de l'ADN synthétisé sur le modèle de l'ARN transformant." *CR Acad Sci*, 1973;276:1625-1628.

10 Beljanski, M. & Plawecki, M., Op cit.

11 Plawecki, M. & Beljanski, M., Op cit.

12 U.S. Patent no. 5413787.

13 Sirsat, M.V. & Shrikhande, S.S. "Histochemical studies on squamous cell carcinomas of the skin arising in burn scars with special reference to histogenesis." *Indian J Cancer*, 1967;3:157-169.

14 James, B. "Mitterrand's cancer: An 11-year secret." *International Herald Tribune*, January 10, 1996: http://www.iht.com/articles/1996/01/10/mitt.t_0.php.

15 James, B., Op cit.

16 James, B., Op cit.

17 Bemis, D.L., et al. "Anti-prostate cancer activity of a beta-carboline alkaloid enriched extract from *Rauwolfia vomitoria*." *Int J Oncol*, 2006 Nov;29(5):1065-73.

18 Bemis, D.L., et al. "Beta-carboline alkaloid-enriched extract from the amazonian rainforest tree Pao pereira suppresses prostate cancer cells." *Soc Integr Oncol*, 2009 Spring;7(2):59-65.

19 Bemis, D.L., et al. *Int J Oncol*, op cit.

20 Bemis, D.L., et al. *Soc Integr Oncol*, op cit.

Index

About the Author

L. Stephen Coles, M.D., Ph.D., is a Visiting Scholar at the University of California at Los Angeles Department of Computer Science and an Assistant Researcher in the Department of Surgery, David Geffen School of Medicine. He co-founded the Los Angeles Gerontology Research Group in 1990, which has met on a monthly basis at UCLA, the University of Southern California, and the California Institute of Technology for the last 19 years. He is a director of the Supercentenarian Research Foundation, which studies persons who have lived to be 110 years or older. Dr. Coles is the author of 129 scientific papers and holds two patents.